CONTENTS

CHAPTER 1

EUROFIT FOR ADULTS

Assessment of health-related fitness

Edited by Pekka Oja and Bill Tuxworth

an[d UKK] Institute for Health Promotion

Committee for the Devel[...]

1995

French edition:

Eurofit pour adultes

Evaluation de l'aptitude physique en relation
avec la santé

ISBN 92-871-2764-6

Publishing and documentation service
Council of Europe
F-67075 Strasbourg Cedex

ISBN 92-871-2765-4
© Council of Europe, 1995
Printed in Finland
Graphic Design and illustrations by Niko Airaksinen
Cover: Atelier de création graphique du Conseil de l'Europe

This handbook was edited by Pekka Oja and Bill Tuxworth on the basis of the work of the Working Party for the CDDS Eurofit Coordinating Group. The members of the Working Party were:

- A. Barabás (Hungary)
- M. Chamorro (Spain)
- B. Ekblom (Sweden)
- H. Levarlet-Joye (Belgium)
- W. van Mechelen (Netherlands)
- P. Oja (Finland), chairman
- B. Tuxworth (U.K.)
- W. Sikorski to the end of 1992 (Poland)

FOREWORD by Professor J. N. Morris

I am happy to welcome Eurofit for Adults. Having been much engaged in the English national fitness survey I can vouch for the hard work, expertise - and good thinking - that have gone into this landmark publication. It should be seen in three contexts.

The manual reflects the growing appreciation of how much physical activity and fitness can contribute to health, well-being and the quality of life in the modern world, and to the elusive goal of 'positive health' that is more than the absence of disease. Physical fitness is surely a manifestation of this - and there is multiplying evidence as well that it can be protective against major disease.

Second, the manual offers something quite new to nations and to communities: scientifically sound and thoroughly practical methods of assessing their own levels of fitness. Baselines of exercise, sporting behaviour and fitness can be measured for the first time using standardized procedures, and programmes tailored to needs and opportunities thus determined. Health gain can be evaluated in participation rates and in subsequent fitness levels, alongside the costs. The methods recommended are valid, repeatable and demonstrably acceptable. Following the widespread use of Children's Eurofit, these methods represent a practical application of exercise physiology and its successful alliance with the concerns of epidemiology. They are "low-tech" of course and do not require elaborate (and expensive) laboratory facilities. The single possible exception is cycle ergometry for aerobic fitness, mainly applicable to individual assessement and the clinical situation, and for which practical, low-cost alternatives are presented.

Third, the manual is a fine example of international scientific collaboration. Hopefully, it will lead to information whereby member countries may both identify the comparative status and needs of sections of their own populations and benefit one another by sharing their experience in seeking to meet those needs.

1995 is something of an annus mirabilis for us. WHO, FIMS, ACSM and CDC (Atlanta), Unesco, all are publishing manifestos to promote physical activity, sport and fitness. These are aimed to counter the enormous waste of human potential for health and well-being evident in the functional incapacities, disease, disability and premature death that are due to the prevalent inactivity and unfitness. The Council of Europe is to be congratulated on its salient contribution to this international initiative.

PREFACE by Daniel Tarchys, Secretary General of Council of Europe

Though more and more people regularly take part in sport and physical recreation, those who do not, and they are numerous, are getting less and less fit to the severe detriment of their health and quality of life. This paradox led the Conference of European Ministers responsible for Sport, meeting in Reykjavik in 1989, to utter an alarm call about adult fitness levels. In response, the Committee for the Development of Sport (CDDS), through its research network and Eurofit experts, has prepared this set of general fitness tests for adults. It is based on the same philosophy, and often uses the same tests, as those in the Eurofit tests for children, endorsed by the Committee of Ministers of the Council of Europe in 1987.

In thanking all those researchers from over 20 member states who have prepared, experimented and agreed these tests, I heartily recommend them to all those - including professionals in fitness centres - who work or who have responsibility in this area; whether they come from sport, public health or education. They are the basic tools, providing essential information for exercise prescription and the foundation for promoting healthy physical activity.

A common and determined effort to use these tests will help initiate a reversal of the dramatic slide in average fitness levels amongst our populations; three hundred million people, of whom the majority lead sedentary lives.

ACKNOWLEDGEMENT

The Eurofit Coordination Group and its Working Party gratefully acknowledge the technical and clerical help the Urho Kaleva Kekkonen Institute for Health Promotion Research (UKK Institute) has provided throughout the process of developing this handbook. This has included the textprocessing of more than a few versions of the manuscript and their delivery, many times in a rush. Special thanks are due to Mrs. Raija Tulimäki, the secretary of the institute, who has efficiently and diligently taken care of all these operations. Also highly appreciated is the generous support and warm hospitality that the Centre d'Alt Rendiment (CAR), the Hungarian University of Physical Education, the Department of Health Science of the Vrije Universiteit of Amsterdam and the UKK Institute have offered in organizing the various meetings of the groups.

INTRODUCTION

This manual presents methods and procedures for the field assessment of fitness among adults, with special emphasis on aspects of fitness or physical capacity related to health. It is intended to be used widely throughout the member states of the Council of Europe for purposes ranging from research to describe and monitor the status of populations, giving vital information for strategy and promotion in public health, recreational provision and education, to counselling and exercise prescription for individuals.

Because of the need for versatility, not only in the ways in which the assessments may be used, but also in the range of ages and conditions of people of both sexes who may be tested, it is a collection of approved tests with alternatives for some key fitness aspects.

Also presented are guidelines for the assessment by questionnaire of physical activity, attitudes to exercise including perceived barriers, contextual health-related behaviours and other information. All or part of such information is an essential complement to the measurement of fitness in the variety of applications referred to above.

The need for a health-related fitness test battery for adults was first presented and approved at the 6th Eurofit Seminar held in Izmir, Turkey in 1990. Based on this initiative the CDDS founded the Eurofit Coordination Group and subsequently its Working Party with the remit to develop a Eurofit test battery for adults. The Working Party with the guidance of the Coordination Group has prepared the manuscript in working meetings and through written contributions by the members. More detailed description of the work of these two groups is given in Appendix 1.

The authors acknowledge and draw attention to the fact that the proposed test battery is by no means a complete, or even less so, a final set of tests. Much more knowledge and experience is needed to establish a definitive test battery which validly and reliably assesses all health-related aspects of fitness, and which is practical to administer in ordinary circumstances for populations at large. However, given the rapidly increasing understanding of the importance of physical activity and good function as health enhancing factors, it is imperative to develop working tools such as the Eurofit test battery, even if imperfect, to support the promotion of sport and physical activity. Therefore, the member countries are invited to apply the battery in a spirit of exploration and experimentation in order to further develop and improve the means of assessing the fitness and health needs of Europeans. Likewise, the future of Eurofit for Adults needs continuing support from all relevant sections of the Council of Europe in order to provide channels for communication between, and monitoring and researching by interested parties throughout Europe.

CHAPTER 1

EUROFIT FOR ADULTS EXPLAINED

Aim and objectives

Eurofit for Adults is a test battery designed for the assessment of health-related fitness. Its general objective is to promote the health, functional capacity and well-being of individuals and populations by providing a tool for the assessment and evaluation of those aspects of fitness which are associated with health.

Purpose

The Eurofit for Adults test battery is designed for the following purposes:
- assessing the status of health-related fitness of individuals, communities, sub-populations and populations
- evaluating the levels of health-related fitness in relation to standard population norms and when possible to criterion values
- providing a knowledge base and facilitating actions aimed at promoting health-related fitness and physical activity

Target population

The primary target group for health-related fitness assessment by Eurofit for Adults is the working-age adult population, ie. from approximately 18, or younger to 65 years of age. Many of the individual tests are likely to be applicable also for most healthy and functionally independent elderly people over the age of 65, but special considerations, which are outside the scope of this manual, need to be taken into account when the battery is applied to elderly populations at large.

Nature and content

Eurofit for Adults is designed to be practical and applicable under conditions available in ordinary communities. It is basically a field test battery in that it does not require a purpose-built space or laboratory equipment, but it can be administered in gymnasiums, sports halls or other similar multipurpose spaces with a minimum of measuring devices and instruments. Although the Eurofit test battery has been designed to be used in simple community settings, its proper administration requires specially trained personnel with proficiency in the testing procedures, understanding of the rationale and interpretation of each test and appreciation for strict standardization of the testing procedures and conditions. Professionals in physical education, education and health care have optimal basic qualifications.

As summarized elsewhere (Chapter 3), research evidence indicates with varying degrees of certainty that lack of physical activity and fitness are associated with obesity, osteoporosis, back problems, cardiovascular diseases, disorders of carbohydrate and lipid metabolism and some psychosocial problems. Most of the respective physiological functions are responsive to acute and chronic physical activity in that the activity acts as a functionally healthy challenge to the system.

The characteristics and functions that are indicative of health or disease states are either morphological or functional. The important morphological characteristics are body composition, bone strength, joint mobility and tissue elasticity, and muscle mass. Cardiovascular function and carbohydrate and lipid metabolism are the key health-related functions. Neuromuscular function is associated with susceptibility to falls, which in turn is directly related to bone fractures, especially in osteoporotic skeletal sites.

The three principal dimensions of health-related fitness are aerobic, musculoskeletal and motor fitness. The associated functions can be characterized by assessing measurable abilities such as cardiorespiratory power and endurance, muscular strength and power, joint mobility and postural control. Body composition is both an important health-related characteristic and a relatively easy quality to assess under non-laboratory conditions, and so represents a especially relevant item for health-related fitness assessment.

Basic concepts

Physical fitness has been defined as "the ability to perform physical work satisfactorily". Often physical fitness refers to performance in athletics and sports. In that context fitness is distinctly task-specific with the aim of maximizing the components of fitness that are central for the sports task in question.

More generally, physical fitness refers to the muscular work needed in one's occupation, in daily tasks and for active leisure time pursuits. For most individuals in the developed countries little muscular effort is usually needed in work and other necessary daily activities. In this context fitness refers to general functional adequacy to withstand physical challenges without overstrain.

It has been noted that even with the generally decreasing physical demands of modern occupations, the work capacity of ageing workers decreases to a critical level if there are no fitness promoting physical activities during leisure time. In later years sufficient functional capabilities not only enable continuing enjoyment of many leisure pursuits but also become fundamental to the maintenance of functional independence and social integrity. Good physical fitness is therefore an indispensable component of overall well-being among the middle-aged and elderly.

Health is a human condition with physical, social and psychological dimensions. Within the concept recently introduced by the World Health Organization, health is a positive phenomenon with emphasis on the individual and societal potential for a full life. Health is a resource for everyday life, not a goal of life in itself. Accordingly, health is a continuum of states encompassing not only the absence of illness but also, and just as importantly, capacities to respond to the challenges encountered in everyday life and resources for the full realization of one's life potential. In this context health includes the functional capabilities necessary for a satisfying and full life.

Health-related fitness can therefore be seen as a set of capabilities conducive to good health in its broadest sense. Capabilities are combinations of individual traits and abilities. The traits in general are genetically determined. Abilities refer to an individual's competence to perform a given muscular task. In the context of health-related fitness both the traits and the abilities are important. While traits are to some extent adaptive to physical activity and training, abilities are usually more sensitive in reflecting changes in physical activity. Therefore, with respect to the assessment of health-related fitness, the abilities in particular lend themselves to meaningful assessment.

It should be emphasised that a person exercising regularly may have an unexpectedly poor result in a particular test due to a low genetic predisposition. Despite that, he or she may well be more physically fit in terms of state of training than the result of the test would indicate. It appears that the important determinant of health-related fitness is the amount and type of exercise. However, since there are today no reliable simple methods for assessing the level of training status, measures of capacity or performance have to suffice. These measures are entirely appropriate as indices of functional adequacy to perform specific tasks in everyday life. The prime usefulness of tests of physical capacities is in recording present status as a marker for monitoring change rather than to classify the fitness of individuals.

Physical Activity and Physical Fitness

Whereas measures of physical capacities or fitness may be of value in their own right, more often they are most useful when they can be interpreted in the context of life-style information about the individual or populations concerned. This information may be complementary to the measures of fitness, or indeed be the major focus of an investigation.

Whereas the value of fitness per se to health has been supported strongly by recent work, (see Chapter 3) almost certainly this is because the measures of fitness reflect participation in physical activity of a type likely to promote good health. The universal consensus anyway, is that the effective strategy to improve the health of an individual or a population is by promoting physical activity, rather than by focusing on fitness levels.

Physical Fitness and Health Promotion

The assessment of fitness must be seen as a descriptive and diagnostic tool within the broad context of the promotion of behavioural change for better health, and not as an end in itself. It is beyond the scope of this manual to set out how the information gained may be used, alongside all the other relevant considerations, to prescribe suitable exercise for individuals, counsel them and motivate them to modify aspects of their lifestyle, and to help them to understand the health gain which can be achieved. These, however, are the ultimate purposes to which testing, if used with sensitivity and understanding, can make a most important contribution, especially in ensuring that the recommended exercise is appropriate, effective, suitable and safe.

CHAPTER 2

BACKGROUND

Historical background to Eurofit

A seminar in Paris in 1978, set up by the Committee for the Development of Sport of the Council of Europe, marked the beginning of work on the Eurofit project. This initiative arose from a growing concern among member nations with regard to the physical fitness of children, given the dramatic changes in lifestyle that have accompanied post-war developments in personal transportation and home-based leisure (car usage and television). More positively it was compatible with the Council of Europe's "Sport for All" policy, a cultural objective implying that no citizen of Europe, particularly the young, should be denied the pleasure and fulfilment of active recreation.

A provisional manual was produced and widely distributed in 1983, and after extensive trials in member states, a revised version was agreed in 1986 and published in 1988. The Committee of Ministers formally recommended the Eurofit Tests to member states in May 1987 (Recommendation No R(87)9). More than 4000 manuals, including the second revised edition of 1993, have been distributed to 25 nations many of whom have produced their own language versions.

While work with the children's Eurofit continues, the interest of the Committee for the Development of Sport has now been directed by the Eurofit coordinating group to the need for a similar approach to providing accredited and standardised methods for the assessment of adult fitness. Discussions on this proposal began at the sixth Eurofit seminar in Turkey in 1990, where delegates from all represented nations expressed their enthusiasm for such a project and their accord as to its objectives. These were the measurement and monitoring of fitness capacities related to positive health. It was clearly the will of the seminar that health should be defined not just as absence of disease but should include the ability to participate in an active lifestyle and retain functional independence into old age.

The coordinating group from 10 countries represents the interests and involvement of the majority of the 38 states now comprising the Council of Europe. It is clear that, while priorities will differ for obvious reasons, not least economic and political upheaval, in

9

different countries, all countries recognize the importance of regular physical activity to physical, mental and social well-being.

The need for a test battery of health-related fitness for adults

The health-related and functional benefits of physical activity and fitness, and the detailed objectives and applications of Eurofit for Adults are described more fully elsewhere in this manual. This introduction briefly points up the developments in society, nature of employment, education, medicine and public health which give a background to the current interest in physical activity and fitness.

Advances in science, technology and medicine have produced profound changes in the nature of living in those countries that have been able to benefit from them. Infectious diseases are no longer a major cause of death in "developed" countries, nor is infant mortality; public sanitation is vastly improved, nutrition better understood and food more plentiful; machines have almost entirely replaced human muscle power at the workplace and largely so in the home. The improvements in public transport and the rapid growth in car ownership have dramatically increased the mobility of individuals, in turn reducing the need to use muscle power to get about. Television in the home is the principal recreation of the majority of Europeans.

While these developments have in the main improved health, life expectation at birth having increased dramatically over the last few decades, they have also brought with them an upsurge in degenerative diseases, especially heart disease. Associated with these modern epidemics is a prevailing sedentary way of life. In other words the very benefits in labour-saving, transport and entertainment at the press of a switch, constitute a direct health risk unless compensated for by some form of regular exercise. Recent research has added to previous knowledge from epidemiological studies that low activity is associated with cardiovascular and other diseases of epidemic proportion and is highly prevalent (for more detailed discussion see Chapter 3).

In developed countries many more people are living at least two decades beyond retirement and ostensibly they are in better medical health than in earlier times. However, population surveys show that their physical capacity to enjoy a full and independent life into old age is of a very low order. For example, osteoporosis is rife among older, postmenopausal women, producing a very high incidence of disabling and often irreparable hip fractures, to which poor muscle strength, power and coordination, also contribute. In Europe's aging populations, approaching 1/4 of whose inhabitants will be over the age of 65 by the end of the century, this is one of today's more important health challenges.

Indeed, the contribution of physical activity and fitness to health, to quality of life and self esteem, means that the promotion of exercise is at the very core of positive public health strategy in modern society.

The use of agreed, standardised fitness measures will allow the monitoring of the condition of populations and the identification of the most needful sub-groups and individuals. Together with information on physical activity and other health related behaviour, and over time with morbidity and also mortality statistics, they will provide knowledge for the better understanding of the interrelationship of health and lifestyle. In this way the resources of health education may be most efficiently targeted at those people most likely to benefit.

Physical Activity and the Environment

In a crowded modern world it is vital that the promotion of sport and exercise should be compatible with environmental and public health concerns. This has not always been seen to be the case. However, participation in active recreation can flourish in ways which complement these concerns. Indeed the Council of Europe's "Sport for All" together with the World Health Organisation's "Healthy Cities 2000" campaigns are directed at improving both the quality of the lives of people and the surroundings in which they live.

While active leisure-time recreation and sport must be the focus of the promotion of physical activity, it is also important to emphasise the ways in which simple exercise such as walking and cycling can benefit both the health of individuals and the quality of the environment. For example, the provision of cycle ways in urban communities and the pedestrianisation of town centres not only improves safety and reduces traffic pollution but also promotes daily physical activity. In this sense fitness is a "green" issue.

References

Eurofit 1993. Handbook for the EUROFIT tests of Physical Fitness. Second edition. Council of Europe, Committee for the Development of Sport, Strasbourg.

CHAPTER 3

THE HEALTH-RELATED AND FUNCTIONAL BENEFITS OF PHYSICAL ACTIVITY AND FITNESS

It is becoming increasingly evident that appropriate physical activity, and hence good fitness, can make a major contribution to the public health of developed nations. Large segments of populations exhibit some life-style related disease risk factors. From the public health point of view, individuals with a few low to moderate risk factor levels can perhaps benefit most from healthy life-style including physical activity. Furthermore, physical inactivity is probably the most prevalent modifiable health risk factor in western populations. Moreover, physical activity has many favourable effects on other risk factors. These observations support the emphasis of moderate to low risk rather than high risk modification strategy in the prevention of diseases, i.e. small changes in several risk factors by a large number of people have the greatest influence on public health.

Physical fitness has been traditionally linked with performance in athletics and sports and to some specialized occupations (e.g. fire-fighters and rescue workers). Highly specific performance-related fitness profiles and respective test batteries have been developed and are widely used in connection with athletic and sport training and as occupational screening and monitoring tools.

Health-related fitness comprises, by definition, those aspects of fitness that are related to health. In developing the health-related fitness concept it is imperative to specify the fitness-health relationships on which the concept is based. Given the versatile and profound physiological and structural challenge that exercise exerts on the human body, it is to be expected that health-related fitness should include many distinct dimensions related to specific aspects of health. These dimensions often coincide with those of performance-related fitness, but may differ in the degree to which they are necessary or desirable.

This chapter examines briefly the available research evidence linking exercise and fitness to health. Since in-depth analysis is outside the scope of this handbook, this chapter is more of a summary of reviews than a systematic examination of original research. Fortunately numerous excellent recent overviews on exercise, fitness and health are available and provide a sound basis for this discussion.

In 1988 the first international consensus symposium on "Exercise, Fitness and Health" was held in Toronto. The purpose was to examine critically the research evidence dealing with the interrelationship between exercise, fitness and health and to formulate an expert consensus statement on the current state of knowledge. This symposium was followed by another similar meeting in 1992 in which the earlier consensus was updated based on new evidence. The published consensus statement and the proceedings of the first (Bouchard et al. 1991) and the second (Bouchard et al. 1994) symposium form the primary knowledge base of the following views. Other recent reviews (Fentem et al. 1988, Vuori 1991, Royal College of Physicians of London 1991, ACSM 1992, Fentem 1992, Pescatello & DiPietro 1993, Morris 1994, Haskell 1994), editorials (Gloag 1992, Gurfman 1993), position statements (CDCP & ACSM 1993) and individual original studies (Sandvik et al. 1993, Paffenbarger et al. 1993, Hambrecht et al. 1993, Lakka et al. 1994) provide further support to the Toronto consensus conclusions.

Recently the potential of physical activity as a health enhancing behaviour has been examined and recognized by several international bodies including the World Health Organization, Fédération Internationale de Médecine Sportive, the American College of Sports Medicine and the Council of Europe. One of the major current projects of CDDS, the Significance of Sport for Society, focuses on physical activity and health as a way to contribute to the European well-being. This project has provided, based on critically assessed scientific knowledge, ministerial recommendations on how to promote health-related sport and physical activity in European countries.

Functional and prophylactic effects of physical activity and training

Table 1(see p. 16-17) summarizes the evidence regarding the functional and health effects of chronic physical activity and training. These are categorized according to the target biological system and with respect to functional adaptation and alterations in the development of disease states. The latter focuses on prophylactic rather than therapeutic and rehabilitative effects. The linkage of functional and prophylactic effects of exercise allows one to relate the evidence not only to disease, but also to the positive end of the health continuum.

Functional adaptation

Abundant research data from well-controlled studies describes the range and complexity of functional adaptations to chronic physical activity. As shown in Table 1 the various cardiovascular, pulmonary, metabolic, neural and tissue adaptations to activity are well understood, while immune, digestive, cognitive and psychological responses at present are less so. Most of the functional adaptations can be considered as conducive to improved quality of life by providing functional reserves above the physical demands of daily life and enabling fulfilling physically active leisure pursuits to be undertaken and enjoyed.

Prophylactic effects

The many well-controlled epidemiological studies indicate, almost without exception, that physical activity protects against **coronary heart disease**. The risk of coronary heart disease is about twice as high in the least active individuals as compared to the most active ones. Results are also consistent with respect to blood pressure in that physical activity and fitness are inversely related to the development of hypertension, and endurance training reduces the resting blood pressure. There is evidence to suggest that regular physical activity may be protective also against atherosclerosis and stroke.

Increasing evidence suggests that weight-bearing exercise strengthens **bone** and attenuates age-dependent bone loss. These changes in turn can decrease the risk of osteoporotic fractures. Senile bone fractures are often the clinical manifestation of osteoporotic bone loss and they occur as a consequence of falls. Many physiological systems including muscular, neural and cognitive, determine susceptibility to falls. However, the evidence linking physical activity and bone fractures via these mechanisms is as yet inconclusive. Studies indicate that physical activity strengthens both the vertebrae and the intervertebral discs and that exercise rehabilitation programmes may be beneficial in the treatment of low back pain, but the role of physical activity and trunk muscle strength and flexibility in the prevention of back pain needs further studies.

Obesity results from the mismatch between energy intake and energy expenditure. Physical activity is likely to prevent, and inactivity to contribute to, the development of obesity. Further prospective studies are needed to clarify the complex relationships. The effects of exercise are most beneficial in moderate overweight though the threshold and degree of health risk associated with relative weight, adiposity and body shape need further study and clarification. The implications for exercise strategy are that it should be directed to prevention of the development of obesity and to treatment of moderate overweight.

Table 1. Effect of physical activity and training on biological functions and respective disease states: summary of research evidence

Biological system	Functional adaptation to physical activity and training		Prophylactic or moderating effect of physical activity and training	
	Function	Evidence[1]	Disease	Evidence[1]
1. Cardiovascular	Stroke volume↑, $\dot{V}O_2$max↑	+++	Atherosclerosis	+
	Total blood volume↑	+++	Coronary heart disease	+++
	Vascular transport capacity↑	+++	Stroke	+
	Fibrinolysis↑, platelet aggregability↓	+	Blood pressure	+++
2. Pulmonary	Total lung capacity, small↑	+++	Chronic lung disease	?
3. Skeletal muscle	Maximum power output↑	+++	Neuromuscular disorders	?
	Capacity to sustain forces and power↑	+++	(Bone fractures subsequent to falls)	+
	Maintenance of muscle mass in the elderly↑	+		
4. Connective tissue	Strength↑	++	Osteoarthritis	?
	Metabolic activity↑	++	Osteoporosis	++
			(Bone fractures subsequent to falls)	
			Back pain	+
5. Adipose tissue	Fat mass↓	+++	Moderate obesity	++
	Visceral adipose tissue↓	+++		
6. Carbohydrate metabolism	Glucose uptake capacity of muscle↑	+++	Type II diabetes	++
	Glycogen sparing↑	+++		
7. Lipid and lipoprotein metabolism	Capacity for fat oxidation↑	+++	Atherogenic lipid profile	+++
8. Immune function	Ability of immune system to respond to an immune challenge↑	+	Infections (moderate training)	+
9. Digestive processes	Colonic peristalsis↑, segmentation↓	+	Colon cancer	+

Biological system	Functional adaptation to physical activity and training		Prophylactic or moderating effect of physical activity and training	
	Function	Evidence[1]	Disease	Evidence[1]
10. Nervous system	Neural transport properties and pathway structures↑	+++	(Bone fractures subsequent to falls)	+
11. Cognitive functions	Reaction time↑	+	(Bone fractures subsequent to falls)	+
12. Psycho-social	Self-esteem, self-efficacy and psychological well-being↑	+	Mild to moderate depression↓ Anxiety↓	+ ++

[1]

+++ proven fact or strong evidence: based on consistent findings of large number of well-designed and controlled studies including randomized controlled trials

++ moderate evidence: based on consistent findings of considerable number of observational cross-sectional and follow-up studies

+ some evidence: based on suggestive findings of few observational studies with methodological weaknesses

17

Research results indicate consistently that exercise improves **glucose tolerance** and reduces **insulin response** in individuals with impaired glucose tolerance or early non-insulin dependent diabetes mellitus (Type II). The effect of exercise training on the metabolic control of more severe non-insulin dependent diabetes mellitus is less clear. There is no conclusive evidence that the glycemic control is improved by exercise training in insulin dependent diabetes (Type I).

Well-controlled observational studies and randomized controlled trials show that regular aerobic activity reduces plasma triglycerides and increases high-density lipoprotein cholesterol, especially in men, thus changing the **lipid profile** to a less atherogenic one.

Research evidence of the preventive effects of physical activity and exercise training on other disease states such as viral infections, some highly prevalent cancers and psychological symptoms such as depression and anxiety is beginning to support a beneficial role for exercise, but more studies are needed particularly in the important area of mental health.

Fitness and health

Many of the functional and prophylactic adaptations of the different biological systems presented in table 1 are closely related to each other. For example, above average maximal aerobic power ($\dot{V}O_2$ max) is known to be associated with low risk of **coronary heart disease**. Many of the physiological functions and morphological characteristics that adapt to physical activity can be expressed in terms of respective capabilities and traits, which constitute the dimensions of health-related fitness. Until recently most of the epidemiologic evidence supporting the cardiovascular health benefits of exercise has been based on the interrelationship of physical activity and health. Skinner and Oja have recently reviewed the literature (1994) regarding the relation between fitness and health. The following is a short summary of their observations.

Body fatness has health implications due to its association with increased risk for hyperlipidemia, hypertension, coronary heart disease and diabetes. Not only total fatness but also the pattern of fat distribution is important. The abdominal visceral fat deposition appears to be particularly critical due to its association with complications in lipoprotein, glucose and insulin metabolism. The fatness-related risk factor profile, particularly that of men, can be markedly improved by exercise training.

The age-related **loss of bone mineral** may lead to osteoporotic bone in later years of life, particularly among women. This increases the risk of fractures, of which especially those of the femur and spine are becoming a significant public health problem in industrialized countries. Considerable evidence shows that bone strength can be increased up to early adulthood and the bone loss can be attenuated throughout the adult years with appropriate physical activity and exercise accompanied by proper diet. Several epidemiological studies indicate that hip fractures are approximately twice as common among inactive persons as among their active controls. This may be due to weaker bones with less resistance to impact caused by falls, and poorer postural control leading to increased risk of falling.

Research into the health benefits of muscular fitness has focused on the aetiology of **low back problems**. Available literature suggests that low levels of strength and endurance of the trunk and supportive muscles may be associated with the development of low back problems. The evidence concerning the causal relations is, however, inconclusive. More research is needed to confirm these relationships and in particular to specify the relative role of extensors and flexors and the relative importance of muscular strength and endurance.

The strength and endurance of the limbs appear to have little relationship to the aetiology and management of specific diseases. However, good muscular performance in general can profoundly improve the **functional freedom and independence** and the overall health of ageing individuals. There is good evidence to show that the trainability of skeletal muscle is preserved in both healthy and frail older adults.

Flexibility may have health implications particularly with regard to **back, hip, neck and shoulder** function. Several observational cross-sectional studies have found that poor thoracic and lumbar mobility is related to an increased risk of back problems. However, more convincing evidence is needed for firm conclusions about the role of spinal mobility in back health. Some of the potential benefits may be compromised by the increased risk of back problems in certain types of activities. Unlike other physical capacities high values, i.e. hypermobility, may also have unfavourable implications for joint health and function.

Motor abilities such as speed and agility appear to have minor importance with respect to the development of diseases. On the other hand, as already mentioned, poor gait and balance are among the risk factors that predispose older individuals to falls leading to bone fractures. There is some evidence to suggest that **postural** control is related to musculoskeletal health by promoting spinal health and by decreasing the risk of falls, especially among the elderly.

Cardiovascular health and diseases have been the focus of most research studying the interrelationships of exercise, fitness and health. It has been consistently shown that not only physical activity but also **aerobic fitness** have important health promoting effects with respect to atherosclerosis and coronary heart disease in particular. These effects appear to be partially independent and partially mediated through the effects on hypertension, non-insulin dependent diabetes and obesity. Some recent results suggest that a moderate level of aerobic fitness provides most of the attainable benefit. For example, Blair et al (1989) showed in a large prospective study that there was a negative relation, independent of other risk factors, between the performance time on treadmill and all-cause and cardiovascular death. More recent findings by the same group reaffirm this association and indicate that it applies to both healthy and chronically ill individuals (Blair et al. 1993).

As indicated in table 1 physical activity and exercise affect carbohydrate and lipid metabolism and the respective disease states in many ways. The resulting metabolic consequences are closely linked with other disease states, in particular the different manifestations of atherosclerosis, hypertension and obesity. It is possible that the metabolic adaptations to exercise explain most of these effects on disease states. Therefore, it would be extremely valuable to have a fitness measure, which would adequately reflect these metabolic responses to training. So far no such measure has been devised.

In summary, considering both the functional and morphological adaptations to chronic physical activity and exercise and their effects on the respective disease states, certain morphological traits and musculoskeletal, motor, aerobic and possibly metabolic abilities can be identified as the important dimensions of fitness, which relate specifically to the health status of adult populations. These dimensions take into account both the positive and negative poles of the health continuum and thus reflect health in its widest context.

References

ACSM 1992. Medicine and Science in Sports and Exercise. Official Journal of The American College of Sports Medicine 24(6) Supplement.

U.S.Centers for Disease Control and Prevention and American College of Sports Medicine. 1993. Summary statement – workshop on physical activity and public health. Sports Med Bull 28(4):7.

Blair SN, Kohl WH III, Paffenbarger RSJr, Clark DG, Cooper KH, Gibbons LW. 1989. Physical fitness and all–cause mortality: a prospective study of healthy men and women. JAMA 262:2395–2401.

Blair SN, Kohl HV, Barlow CE. 1993. Physical activity, physical fitness, and all–cause mortality in women: do women need to be active? J Am Coll Nutr 12(4):368–371.

Bouchard C, Shephard RJ, Stephens T, Sutton JR, McPherson BD, eds. 1990. Exercise, Fitness, and Health. A Consensus of Current Knowledge. Human Kinetics, Champaign, Illinois.

Bouchard C, Shephard RJ, Stephens T, McPherson BD, eds. 1994. Physical Activity, Fitness and Health. Human Kinetics, Champaign, Illinois.

British Medical Association 1992. Cycling: towards health and safety. Oxford University Press 10–28, 111–31, Oxford.

Fentem PH, Bassey EJ, Turnbull NB. 1988. "The New Case for Exercise". Health Education Authority, London.

Fentem PH. 1992. Exercise in prevention of disease. Br Med Bull 48(3):630–650.

Gloag D. 1992. Exercise, fitness, and health. Br Med J 305:377–378.

Gurfman GD. 1993. The health benefits of exercise. N Engl J Med 328(8):574–576.

Hambrecht R, Niebauer J, Marburger C, Grunze M, Kälberer B, Hauer K, Schlierf G, Kübler W, Schuler G. 1993. Various intensities of leisure time physical activity in patients with coronary artery disease: effects on cardiorespiratory fitness and progression of coronary atherosclerotic lesions. J Am Coll Cardiol 22:468-477.

Haskell WL. 1994. Health consequences of physical activity: understanding and challenges regarding dose-response. Med Sci Sports Exerc 26(6):649-660.

Lakka TA, Venäläinen JM, Rauramaa R, Salonen R, Tuomilehto J, Salonen JT.1994. Relation of leisure-time physical activity and cardiorespiratory fitness to the risk of acute myocardial infarction in men. N Engl J Med 330:1549-1554.

Morris JN. 1994. Exercise in the prevention of coronary heart disease: today's best buy in public health. Med Sci Sports Exerc 26(7):807-814.

Paffenbarger RS, Hyde RT, Wing AI, Lee I-M, Jung DI, Kampert JB. 1993. The association of changes in physical activity level and other lifestyle characteristics with mortality among men. N Engl J Med 328:538-45.

Pescatello LS, DiPietro L.1993. Physical activities in older adults: An overview of health benefits. Sports Med 15(6):353-364.

Royal College of Physicians of London. 1991. Medical aspects of exercise: benefits and risks. London: RCP.

Skinner JS, Oja P. 1994. Laboratory and field tests for assessing health-related fitness. In: Bouchard C, Shephard RJ, Stephens T, McPherson BD, eds. Physical Activity, Fitness and Health. Human Kinetics, Champaign, Illinois 160-179

Vuori I 1991. Sport for all in health and disease. In: Oja P,Telama R, eds. Sport for all. Elsevier Science Publishers B.V. 33-44.

CHAPTER 4

DIMENSIONS OF EUROFIT FOR ADULTS

Based on the interrelationships of physical activity and fitness and their contributions to positive health, the principal dimensions of health-related fitness for adults are:

      1. aerobic fitness
      2. musculoskeletal fitness
      3. motor fitness
      4. body composition

Aerobic fitness

Aerobic fitness is a key component of health-related fitness. Maximal oxygen uptake ($\dot{V}O_2$ max) is the objective measure of the power of the aerobic chain consisting of respiratory, cardiovascular and metabolic functions. It reflects the training status and the level of habitual physical activity of an individual within genetically determined limits. Directly or indirectly assessed $\dot{V}O_2$ max has been extensively used in the study of fitness-health relationships and it has been shown consistently to be linked with morbidity, mortality and several disease risk factors. Aerobic fitness is the single most important dimension of overall functional fitness needed for everyday physical demands.

Musculoskeletal fitness

Musculoskeletal fitness consists of muscular strength and endurance and flexibility. The strength and endurance of the trunk muscles is the most important aspect of muscular fitness with respect to health. Since the specific importance of trunk flexors and extensors or other muscle groups involved in trunk function is not known, the trunk musculature as a whole must be considered. Furthermore, little is known about the specific health implications of strength vs. endurance and dynamic vs. static contraction. Therefore the health-related assessment of trunk muscular performance must take all these aspects into account.

While there appears to be no specific and direct health consequence of the muscular performance of the extremities, sufficient strength and endurance of arms and legs is imperative in retaining proficient functioning in most daily activities especially with advancing age. As with the trunk musculature the functional implications concern the gross performance of the arm and leg musculature.

The health-related interest in flexibility focuses on trunk and shoulder mobility. Again no specific joint or section of the spinal-hip complex can be singled out as more important than others, but it is the functional mobility of the entire chain that is of importance. This gross mobility includes not only the mobility of the involved joints as determined by their ligaments and capsules, but also the movement allowed by the adjoining muscles and tendons. Although good trunk mobility is thought to be conducive to back health, joint laxity may also entail a risk for joint health.

Motor fitness

Motor fitness is important in many sporting events but it also has health implications. These concern particularly those motor abilities that determine susceptibility to falls and the consequent bone fractures and back problems. It is apparent that postural and movement control of the whole body are central abilities in this respect. These abilities consists of complex combinations of neuromuscular, sensory and proprioceptive functions and are difficult to assess. However, measures of whole body balance and coordination provide an impression of certain aspects of these functions and they can be assessed by relatively simple field tests.

Other motor abilities such as speed and agility are perhaps less critical with respect to the health and function of adult and ageing population. Reaction time and speed of small muscles, for example, are important abilities for manual dexterity, but there appears to be a large margin of safety for sufficient functioning in ordinary living conditions.

Body composition

The most important aspects of body composition are body fatness and fat distribution. Body fatness is expressed by the relative proportion of fat weight within the total body weight. It can be estimated with reasonable accuracy by simple measures such as the thickness of subcutaneous fat and is reflected by body mass index (BMI). The truncal-abdominal fatness and in particular the visceral fatness are thought to be the most important health-related features of fat distribution. While there are no direct methods for their assessment outside the laboratory, the simple ratio of waist to hip circumference provides an indirect impression of this distribution.

Physical activity and health status

Health-related life-style and health status are integral parts of health promoting fitness assessment. Previous and current physical activity and exercise pattern directly serve the evaluation of the test results and the consequent exercise prescription and counseling. Information on unhealthy habits such as tobacco smoking, excessive alcohol consumption and poor diet, complement the data on exercise behaviour and allow for holistic life-style counselling.

Self-assessed health status and disease history provide necessary additional information for the administration of the tests, interpretation of the results and guidance for exercise. Safety is a necessary quality of any test battery designed to be used for population fitness assessment. Therefore a procedure for the evaluation of health status should be an integral part of all fitness testing programmes and settings. Extensively tested self-assessment methods like the PAR-Q and its modifications (Chisholm et al 1975, Chisholm et al 1978, Thomas et al 1992, see references for Chapter 6) are available for this purpose. More objective assessment of health status and disease risk factors allows clinically oriented evaluation of exercise potential, risks for exercise and targets for health behaviour changes. These measures are optional and they should be designed and implemented in cooperation with medical expertise.

In summary the basic structure of the Eurofit test battery for adults is as follows:

Dimension	Component
1. Aerobic fitness	maximal aerobic power
2. Musculoskeletal fitness	a. muscular strength and endurance
	b. flexibility
3. Motor fitness	a. balance
	b. speed
4. Body composition	a. body fatness
	b. fat distribution
Physical activity and health status	-

CHAPTER 5

THE EVALUATION OF FITNESS TEST RESULTS - WHAT DO THE OUTCOMES SIGNIFY?

What criteria are there?

Before proceeding to the evaluation of individual test results, and interpreting them in terms of personal or population states, it is necessary to consider what criteria can be applied.

At present, there are no precise formulae or indices which describe how much physical fitness, or physical activity is required for optimum health gain. Despite well-known prescriptions for exercise "to maintain and develop cardiorespiratory fitness", as yet there is little secure knowledge quantifying the dosage for health. This applies even to the best documented benefit, i.e. in protecting against coronary heart disease. Still less is known about exercise dosage for other health benefits - bone strengthening and reduction of osteoporosis, the management of disease, such as chronic bronchitis or depression; or the retention of flexibility into old age. However increasing research interest in the dose-response relationships between physical activity, fitness and health benefits is rapidly providing a more secure knowledge base for exercise prescription.

More positively, however, as Chapter 3 makes clear, there is very strong evidence indeed that physically active people are healthier in ways particularly relevant to the morbidity and mortality profile of developed countries. Some major studies propose thresholds of benefit, which can be used to construct provisional criteria. These criteria, based on activity levels or intensities, can in turn be interpreted as requiring adequate levels of fitness to be achievable.

Recently, direct evidence of the reduced all-cause and cardiovascular mortality associated with fitness itself, as measured using well authenticated procedures, gives a basis for proposing "desirable" fitness levels for such health gain. The direction of accumulating evidence suggests that the association of fitness with health is rapidly being established beyond reasonable doubt.

Interpretation

There are two basic approaches to interpreting the results of fitness tests:

By reference scales of established **population norms**: answering the question "where does this particular score lie in the distribution of values in the population?"

and by reference to **criterion values**, i.e. thresholds of reduced risk, "minimum", "desirable", "acceptable" levels etc: answering questions such as "does this score meet the level required for reduced risk of heart disease or other health gain?"

The interpretation of results of fitness tests for performance is relatively simple using either of these approaches. For example, an aspiring marathon runner will need an aerobic fitness score high in the general population distribution for competitive success, above a certain minimum level to complete the course, and above definable levels for different orders of performance. Interpretation for health gain is more complex.

Reference to Population Norms and Distributions

The first approach, that of using reference scales, based on results for representative population samples, allows the formation of distribution percentile categories. The raw score can then be described as eg. "at the 50th percentile", "within the top or bottom quintile" and so on. This sort of classification by quintiles might typically be labelled as "far above average", "above average", "average", "below average" and "far below average".

There are obvious **limitations** arising from this approach, viz:

• The borders of each category are subject to confidence intervals related to the sample size and do not constitute precise divisions.

• Within a population the fitness levels may fluctuate and thus a spurious indication may be given of the change or stability of the individual score.

• The reference scales are specific with regard to geographical region and sociocultural factors. They should be used with caution for populations other than those from which they were formulated. The English and Swedish population norms given in Chapter 6 are based on large random samples and thus provide representative reference values for the respective study populations.

The Use of Value Categories

An additional problem arises when reference scales are used in a qualitative sense, as bases for value categories. Hence, reference scales may typically be divided into five or more categories labelled as "excellent", "good", "average", "poor" and "very poor". This scale ascribes quality merely to status within the population, and does not attempt to explain what benefit or disbenefit is conferred by "good" or "poor" fitness. In this sort of categorisation the assumption will often be made that "average", lying between "good" and "poor" must mean "satisfactory". The fallacy of such an assumption is obvious - unless it can otherwise be shown that "average" levels of fitness within the population described do in fact confer definable health benefit.

However, people do express an interest in "where they stand" in relation to their peers. This interest has to be recognised, and its often counterproductive outcome - discouragement or complacency - must somehow be deflected or dealt with.

Criterion Values

Criterion values are the most logical yardsticks for interpreting the raw scores from fitness tests in terms of health gain. As already pointed out, these criterion values are not yet established, but for some aspects of fitness, especially aerobic, there are some useful indicators.

Definitions of health range from "absence of disease" to a broader concept embracing quality of life, including the retention of functional capacity for the activities of daily living and recreation in an ageing population. Therefore the question "how much fitness is required for health?" has no single answer. Thus, the proposed criteria for aerobic fitness may relate to both disease protection and functional adequacy, while the direct disease benefit may not be quantifiable in any meaningful way for muscle strength, joint flexibility and so on. The benefits in terms of retention of function may however be easier to specify and to quantify. Body composition may be both directly related to disease risk and also modify functional adequacy.

Criterion values for aerobic fitness

A variety of sources is drawn upon to arrive at an evaluation of the level of aerobic fitness which appears to be desirable for protection from the major cause of premature death in Western civilisations, coronary heart disease (CHD).

Epidemiological studies in general do not classify intensity of physical activity, with the exception of Morris et al's (1980) longitudinal study of 18,000 middle aged male civil servants. The outcome of this study, reinforced over long term observation, was that reported physical activity reaching at least 7.5 kcals/min energy expenditure was the threshold for the health benefit mainly being studied - i.e. substantial protection against CHD. This corresponds to about 1.5 litres/min oxygen uptake (or about 21 ml per kilogram bodyweight per minute in a person weighing 70 kg). For that energy expenditure to be sustained in excess of a few minutes it would have to be no more than about 60-65% of maximal oxygen uptake ($\dot{V}O_2$ max) or 70-75% of maximum heart rate in the average individual. This brings us to a notional $\dot{V}O_2$ max for health benefit of about 32-35 ml/kg/min. (Habitual exertion at the 21 ml/kg/min level would normally entail this order of functional reserve capacity). An important limitation of this approach is that it can only be applied with confidence to the age range of males in Morris et al's study, 40-64 years at outset and observed for approximately 9 years.

A cluster of studies from several developed nations report mean levels of aerobic fitness for men in their fifties as between the high 20s and middle to high 30s (ml/kg/min). From this the general impression could be gained that desirable aerobic fitness levels for cardiovascular health benefit are achieved by between 1/3 and 2/3 of middle aged males in Western populations.

Measured Fitness and Health

Blair et al's (1989) study of measured fitness and all-cause mortality, while showing a clear and substantial association between aerobic fitness and survival, only (in the initial publication) attributed significant benefit to being above the lowest quintile in the aerobic fitness distribution. For women, and to a lesser extent for men, additional benefit accrued from being above the second lowest quintile, but no further benefit was obtained by higher levels of fitness. The upper borders of the bottom and fourth quintiles, were in the 40-49 year old and 50-59 year old men, 32 and 34 ml/kg/min maximal oxygen uptake and 28 and 30 ml/kg/min respectively. For women, they were 23 and 26 ml/kg/min and 21 and 22 ml/kg/min respectively. This appears to suggest a scaling of desirable levels of fitness for health benefit to age and sex. Further person-years of experience and analysis have strengthened the association between fitness and low all-cause mortality. Thus benefit of decreased mortality extends to the top 40% of the fitness distribution. For the age and sex groups discussed above, the mean maximal oxygen uptakes for the top 40% are of the order of 45 and 39 ml/kg/min (5th and 6th decade men) and 33 and 30 ml/kg/min (5th and 6th decade women).

Other studies, most notably by Ekelund et al (1988), strongly support the health benefit of fitness, showing similar advantage of fit over unfit men especially with regard to coronary heart disease, the least fit men being more than 8 times as likely to die of CHD.

Many expert considerations of this issue have been made and from the variety of conclusions or opinions no consensus has yet emerged, particularly as to how fitness for health gain might be graded for age. Given the inevitable decline in physical capacities due to the ageing process itself, it seems unrealistic to set targets based on one absolute level of desirable fitness for all ages. Such a level would be relatively easy to achieve and already more prevalent among younger people, while it might be totally unrealistic for a very large proportion of older people. It would seem sensible to adjust targets in relation to age, and given the decline with age, to set those targets somewhat higher, ie. well above the present-status criterion level, for young and early middle age. In this way any loss, despite continuing activity, over the next decades would still leave them with adequate fitness for necessary daily exertion and ideally a functional reserve for recreation.

A practical approach from the foregoing rationale could be that fitness levels of the order of about 46-52 ml/kg/min $\dot{V}O_2$max in young men decreasing to 35-40 ml/kg/min by the seventh decade might constitute viable and realistic targets. Though information is scantier for women regarding health gain, and health concerns might emphasise different aspects of fitness, equivalent levels for women might be 42-48 ml/kg/min for young women declining to 30-35 ml/kg/min by the seventh decade. This scheme is based on estimates of $\dot{V}O_2$max using walking as the excercise mode. For estimates received from stationary cycling values some 5-10% lower might be appropriate.

However, whatever the targets in health promotion are, great care must be exercised in their use ie. to make sure that they are appropriate for the individual whose potential for improvement must be realistically assessed. Change towards better health via increased functional capacity and lower risk is the objective, and the individual must not be discouraged, especially the individual of low genetic endowment, by remote and seemingly unachievable goals. This applies equally to population reference values, but is more acute with a criterion based approach where a certain level of fitness might be presented as "a necessary minimum" for good health.

Finally, health-related criterion values are not to be confused with diagnostic criteria such as are used in the interpretation of "stress tests" - except in the very broadest sense where the outcome is "diagnostic" of a sedentary lifestyle.

Functional basis for assessing the adequacy of aerobic fitness for health

Functional adequacy may be difficult to define if one considers only young healthy adults. However, in the elderly, minimal needs for self-sufficient mobility and the activities of daily living are much clearer, as are the benefits to quality of life brought by higher levels of physical capacity.

Whatever one's age or sex, if one wishes to retain the ability to get about and perform normal everyday physical tasks, with all the psychological and social advantages that these entail - f'tness to do so must be maintained. Distances do not shorten nor hills become less steep in response to the passing of years. A reserve capacity above minimal needs for recreational activity is increasingly eroded with age unless the regular habit of exercise levels to provoke a compensatory "training effect" is maintained.

In the English national fitness survey report (The sports Council and the Health Education Authority 1992) an approach was used to interpret the results of the aerobic fitness test based on ability to walk at what were considered "normal speeds and gradients". While value judgements had to be made regarding what speeds, durations and gradients comprised appropriate reference tasks, the criteria for achievement were based on objective physiological data from the treadmill test.

It was considered that two levels of walking task were relevant to everyday mobility, at least the less strenuous of which might reasonably be expected to be achievable throughout life by a healthy individual of either sex.

The tasks were:
Ability to walk "comfortably" at 4,7 km/h (approximately 3 mph) on level ground and up a 1:20 (5%) gradient.

The qualification "comfortably" was all important. It meant that the task should be sustainable - not rapidly exhausting, ie. a person could walk at this speed and gradient for more than just a few minutes without fatigue or distress.

For the English survey report, a population generalisation for the ceiling of aerobic work (or "anaerobic threshold") was made as 70% of maximum heart rate. In other words, if an individual's heart rate exceeded 70% of their maximum at the level of expenditure required by the walking task, it was considered that the task was not sustainable.

This approach can easily be applied to show the extent and distribution of functional inadequacy within a population. For example in the English survey a very high proportion of middle-aged and older men (about 45 % aged 50 and 80 % aged 65), and even greater numbers of women (80 % and over 90 % ,respectively) were incapable of the uphill walking task. Those incapable even of comfortable normal paced walking on level ground, were sufficiently numerous to cause serious concern (eg. 30 % of men and 50 % of women aged 60).

33

A functional reference task approach of this nature can be shown to be compatible with other health criteria. It is interesting to note that the more severe task, walking at 4.7 km/h up a 1:20 slope, requires, for the average middle-aged man, an energy expenditure of the order of 7.5 kcal/min (Morris' postulated protective level of exertion). To be achieved aerobically it would require a maximal oxygen uptake of the order of 32-35 ml/kg/min - which again recalls values arrived at from a different perspective in the earlier discussion. Again, for our average sedentary male, the two tasks require oxygen uptakes of about 1 and 1.5 l/min respectively. Considerable interest has been shown in the use of indices to describe aerobic fitness based on heart rate responses to these levels of oxygen uptake (Collins 1990). Similarly, in cycle ergometry the approximately equivalent load to 1.5 l/min $\dot{V}O_2$ (100 Watts) has been used in the rehabilitation of cardiac patients as an indicator for monitoring improvement in exercise tolerance.

An advantage with a functional reference task is that it presents an immediately understandable target to the individual. It is a more appealing and tangible objective to walk a mile in a certain time, say 20 minutes, than to move up l0 percentile points in the population distribution or increase $\dot{V}O_2$max by so many millilitres. It can also directly provide the exercise prescription itself, identifying the level of exercise needed for improvement of fitness. The 2 km walk test provides opportunities for this kind of functional interpretation.

Criterion values for other aspects of fitness

Where muscular strength, endurance and power are concerned, direct health related criteria do not exist in terms of protection from disease. However, with regard to function, useful and meaningful reference values can be derived from studies on older people. For example, thresholds of adequacy in terms of minimal strength or power for rising unaided from a low chair or toilet, or in stair climbing, are available and are described elsewhere (in the discussion of individual test results). For joint flexibility criteria are elusive, the debate concerning validity and interpretation of the "sit-and- reach" test (often referred to as forward or trunk flexion) remain to be unresolved. A functional threshold for limited shoulder joint movement has been proposed, and side bending scores have been shown to associate with indices of back health (Suni et al. 1994).

The interpretation of anthropometry - measurements of height, weight, girths, derived indices such as Body Mass Index (BMI) and waist to hip ratio, and assessment of body fat - rests on the criteria derived from evidence about the nature and health risk of overweight/obesity and of underweight, and the extent to which modifications are feasible or desirable, as discussed in Chapter 3 and again in Chapter 6. Apart from direct health implications, body weight is used in the expression of several fitness indices.

Final note

In the following chapter, at the end of the description and protocol for each test, guidance is given regarding evaluation in two categories. These categories correspond to those already discussed i.e. reference and criterion values. For many of these tests the criterion values do not yet exist or have a very meagre research basis. However, this reflects limited information rather than a weak association with health gain. Consistent associations and hence secure criterion values will emerge from well controlled and organised studies using Eurofit. In this sense Eurofit for adults is a collective European research enterprise.

References

Blair SN, Kohl WH III, Paffenbarger RSJr, Clark DG, Cooper KH, Gibbons LW. 1989. Physical fitness and all–cause mortality: a prospective study of healthy men and women. JAMA 262:2395–2401.

Ekelund L–G, Haskell WL, Johnson JL, Whaley FS, Criqui MH, Sheps DS. 1988. Physical fitness as a predictor of cardiovascular mortality in asymptomatic North American men: the lipid research mortality follow–up study. N Engl J Med 319:1379–1384.

International Union of Biological Sciences. 1990. "Handbook of Methods for the Measurement of Work Performance, Physical Fitness and Energy Expenditure". Collins KI, ed. IUBS, Paris.

Morris JN, Everitt MG, Pollard R, Chave SPW, Semmence AM. 1980. Vigorous exercise in leisure time: protection against coronary heart disease. Lancet ii:1207–1210.

Suni J, Oja P, Laukkanen R, Miilunpalo S, Pasanen M, Vartiainen T–M, Vuori I. 1994. The relation of functional back health with motor, musculoskeletal and cardiorespiratory fitness in adult population. Med Sci Sports Exerc 26(5) (Suppl.):S9 A–14 50 (abstract).

The Sports Council and the Health Education Authority. 1992. Allied Dunbar national fitness survey. A report on activity patterns and fitness levels. Belmont Press, London.

Table 2. Structure of the Adult Eurofit test battery.

DIMENSION	COMPONENT	FACTOR	TEST 1st Priority	TEST 2nd Priority	TEST 3rd Priority
Aerobic fitness	Maximal aerobic power	Maximal aerobic power	2 km walk test or bicycle test or shuttle–run (20 m)		
Musculoskeletal fitness	Muscle strength & endurance	Trunk muscle endurance	Dynamic sit–up		
		Leg muscle power		Vertical jump	
		Arm muscle endurance		Bent arm hang	
		Hand muscle strength			Hand grip
	Flexibility	Trunk flexion	Side bending or Sit & reach		
		Shoulder mobility		Shoulder abduction	
Motor fitness	Balance	Whole body balance	Single leg balance		
	Speed	Hand movement speed			Plate tapping
Anthropometry	Height Weight	Body Mass Index	Weight for height		
	Skinfolds	Sum of X skinfolds	Estimate of body fatness		
	Waist girth Hip girth	Waist–to–hip ratio	Estimate of fat distribution		

Physical activity and health questionnaire

CHAPTER 6

THE EUROFIT TEST BATTERY FOR ADULTS

General recommendations

The test battery

The collection of tests - or more correctly assessments, because there is no 'pass' or 'fail' - comprising Eurofit for Adults, stems from the rationale in Chapters 3 and 4. These chapters reviewed the health benefits of exercise and identified the components of physical fitness of greatest relevance. The proposed tests all represent approved, valid and reliable measures of these components. While the priority accorded to a particular test (.e.g aerobic fitness 1st priority, aspects of motor fitness 2nd or 3rd priority) is generally appropriate, it is recognised that for some individuals or groups a different relative importance may exist (e.g. with regard to the management of certain diseases or ageing-related loss of function). For general purposes however the priority accorded reflects the relative importance of fitness components to health.

The structure of the Eurofit test battery for adults is presented in table 2. The first priority tests include test items for the assessment of aerobic fitness, trunk muscular endurance, and flexibility. Whole body balance is included because of its particular importance for older individuals. Anthropometry, health audit and activity assessment are also integral parts of a comprehensive battery.

For the assessment of aerobic fitness three test options are provided: the 2 km walking test, a cycle ergometer test and the 20 meter endurance shuttle run. All yield a measure of aerobic fitness and can be used as alternatives according to the circumstances of testing.

While two tests of flexibility are included in the first priority listing, this reflects some controversy regarding the status of the more conventional approach ("sit and reach") and differing information needs. When selecting a test for flexibility the chosen test should be that most likely to give the type of information required. Shoulder abduction could well assume first priority status for older individuals.

Within the group of first priority tests, it is recommended that the following comprises the minimum viable battery:

- a test of aerobic fitness
- a test of musculoskeletal fitness
- anthropometry (at least height, weight and waist and hip girths)
- assessment of physical activity and health status

The second priority tests measure the muscular performance of the upper and lower limbs and the shoulder mobility. The link between these fitness factors and health is less clearly evidenced than is the case for the main tests, but since adequate limb performance is critical for proper function in many everyday tasks, especially with increasing age, these tests are recommended to supplement the information given by the first priority tests.

The third priority tests are the hand grip test and the plate tapping test. The health relation of these tests is somewhat more specific in that they reflect functional capabilities of importance for special groups. They are recommended as further optional tests where appropriate. Both are also in the Children's Eurofit battery, and therefore important for tracking studies.

The tests in the battery have been evaluated with respect to their validity, reliability, feasibility and usefulness. Validity refers to both criterion and cross validity. For a test to be reliable it must have good intra- and intertester repeatability. The feasibility of a given test concerns its applicability to population assessment. Other important considerations are suitability for large segments of populations, safety, practicality, modest technical requirements and availability of reference values. The general usefulness reflects qualities such as social acceptability and scientific value. The selected tests have been included in the battery on the condition that they are the most satisfactory available in all or most of these qualities.

Some tests are described at greater length than others. This does not reflect their relative importance. The more detailed instructions are given for tests which are more complex to administer and/or are less well known.

General testing conditions

The value and effectiveness of the Eurofit tests will to a major extent depend on rigorous testing procedures and the degree to which the tester can reassure, encourage and motivate the person being assessed.

The rigour of test procedures depends on the following:

- Careful selection and thorough training of staff.
- Proper sequence, organisation and conduct of each test.
- Maintenance and calibration of equipment.
- Clarity and simplicity of recording results.
- An appropriate environment for the test.

The co-operation and optimum achievement by the person being assessed depends on the following:

- A friendly welcome in a calm, restful environment.
- Arrival in comfortable time for several minutes rest before the tests begin.
- Appropriate information in advance about suitable clothing and pre test requirements regarding eating, drinking, smoking and exercise (see below).
- A full explanation of the nature, duration and purpose of the test, together with any necessary reassurances before each test is performed.
- Encouragement and vigilance regarding the subject's condition, especially towards the end of the exertional tests - in particular aerobic and muscular endurance.
- The tester's credibility (professional, calm, dealing effectively with any equipment problems, able to answer the subject's questions).

Temperature and Ventilation

While strict conditions for temperature, ventilation and humidity cannot be adhered to in a field situation, especially given the climatic and weather variations in member states, it is unwise for the tests to be carried out in uncomfortably cold conditions (less than 15°C) except for walking tests which may be held in colder conditions wearing adequate clothing and with some prior warm-up. Temperatures above 25°C are also unsuitable, and will give adversely affected results, as well as imposing some hazard especially for overweight subjects and those with mild hypertension. Similarly days of high humidity and/or poor air quality should also be avoided for the aerobic fitness tests.

Exertion, Food, Alcohol, Stimulants and Tobacco

As a general recommendation, subjects should be asked to avoid hard exercise and the use of alcohol within 24 hours, and stimulants or tobacco within 2 hours of commencing the entire test battery. These constraints are particularly important not only for a valid outcome but also for the comfort and safety of the subjects during any of the tests requiring muscular exertion.

Sequence of the tests

Any test requiring exertion must be preceded by the required health screening. The sequence in which the tests are performed, unless they are performed on separate occasions, will affect the results and in some cases their acceptability to the subject. It is recommended to begin with the non-exertional tests, i.e. anthropometry, and progress via flexibility, balance and speed of movement (if included) to the tests of muscular strength and endurance. The final test after a suitable rest interval should always be the test of aerobic fitness.

Evaluation of the Test Results

When evaluating results of the tests, two possibilities exist:

First, one can compare within the same subject a score obtained at a certain point in time with a score obtained on a later occasion. Secondly, the individual result can be compared with population reference norms. Particular attention may then be paid to individual results in the lowest quintile of the population distribution and possibly also in the quintile above that. Results falling into these categories may imply deficiencies in functional capability, which may require and be amenable to, improvement. For further discussion of the interpretation of the test results see Chapter 5.

Description of the Tests and Measurements

Aerobic fitness

A choice of three tests is available for the assessment of aerobic fitness, two performance tests and one of aerobic power. Each is well validated and optimally fulfils the requirements of different circumstances of testing.

Thus the **two kilometre walking test** is most suitable for mixed groups of adults. It enables large numbers of people to be tested within the space of a short afternoon or morning, and has proved popular and highly motivating. It also uses walking, the most natural physical activity of all. Like all tests, it needs careful administration and good organisation, but is less demanding of specialised knowledge than the ergometer test. Usually it is carried out out-of-doors.

Of the three, the **ergometer test (cycle)** is probably the most accurate measure of aerobic power and has the advantage of being almost entirely objective i.e. requiring no special motivation or pace judgement. It is a sub-maximal test and allows for continuous surveillance of the subject's responses and condition. It provides entirely comparable and very reliable information for monitoring change in physiological response to progressive, quantified exercise. It is, however, demanding of resources in terms of relatively expensive equipment and administrator time and expertise. It is perhaps the best suited test for an individual appraisal within a counselling session.

The **multi-stage shuttle run** has been re-evaluated for adult use and found to be suitable for testing well motivated groups of relatively active people interested in improving their fitness for participation in sport, e.g. team games. It has an advantage over other walking or running tests (e.g. Cooper) in that it requires little or no pace judgement, the pace being imposed by the electronic "beep". It is, however, a maximal test, and is unsuitable for sedentary, older people or those with locomotive difficulties in running, or where it may be counter-productive for people to compare their performance too obviously

CHAPTER 6

with others. It requires careful, well-organised administration but inexpensive equipment. Several people can be tested together.

While the required expertise in technical or physiological knowledge may differ between the tests, it is important that in all cases, the administering staff are competent and vigilant in their surveillance of every participant's condition, particularly with regard to undue fatigue or distress.

When evaluating the test results in relation to population norms test-specific reference values should be used. Thus, different reference values are given for the walking test and the cycle test, the former being from a Finnish population sample (see p. 45) and the latter from a Swedish population sample (table 3, p. 95). Unfortunately, no population reference values are available for the shuttle-run test.

2-km walking test

Aim

The two kilometer walking test is a brisk walking performance accompanied by simple measurements. It provides direct information on walking fitness (time and heart rate) and can be used to predict maximal oxygen uptake. A population based fitness index can be derived.

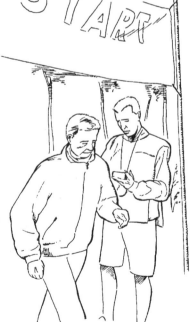

Background

Walking is a comfortable and simple exercise mode for nearly all adults. It is a useful exercise mode for cardiovascular fitness testing due to its simplicity, sufficient physiological loading, safety and social acceptability. A series of studies have shown that the walking test is a valid, reliable and feasible test for healthy adult populations, except for those with very high levels of $\dot{V}O_2$max. It has been designed specifically for field conditions. The test is extensively used in a variety of settings and it has proved to be highly motivating even for sedentary individuals.

Description of the test

The test performance is a brisk (relative to an individual's capacity) 2 km walk on level ground. The test result, either a prediction of $\dot{V}O_2$max or a derived fitness index, is calculated from the time for the 2-km walk, heart rate at the end of the walk, body mass index (kg/m^2), and age.

Conditions for the test

Too hot (>25°C) or too cold (<5°C) ambient temperature will adversely affect performance and the test result as well as introducing a health hazard to some individuals. High humidity and poor air quality should also be avoided. The subject should wear comfortable leisure clothing, good walking shoes or trainers. In order to alleviate the muscle soreness that can often follow the fast walk, stretching exercise for the legs and warm up walk before the test and cool down walk afterwards are recommended.

Procedure

The fitness card is given to the subject before the test, whereupon he/she fills in the identification information (name, age, height, weight) and answers the screening questionnaire. The tester uses this information to decide whether the person can do the test and for the interpretation of the results. Before the test the subject is instructed to warm up for a few minutes. This should include stretching of the legs and a preliminary fast walk of at least 200 metres to try out walking pace, during which the tester should assist the subject. Subjects are started at convenient intervals (30 seconds is usual) and instructed to "walk as fast as possible with an even pace". The performance should be supervised during the walk in order to achieve fast enough but steady walking pace at the finish. A the finish the elapsed time is taken to the nearest second and the heart rate is recorded immediately. The starting, finishing and walking times, as well as the heart rate, are all recorded on the test card. After the test the results are calculated according to the formulas (given in the fitness card) by calculator, tables or using a computer program.

Equipment

* A track with firm and smooth surface on level ground allowing 2 km of continuous walking (eg. a 500 m straight is acceptable). The total distance should be accurate to 5 metres.

* Test cards and fitness cards

* Stopwatch

* Heart rate recorder

* Signs indicating the starting and finishing points

* Weighing scales

* Pocket calculator, calculation tables or computer

Calculations

The fitness index is based on walking time, heart rate, BMI, age and sex. It takes into account the age-dependent decline in population aerobic fitness yielding a value which can be compared with age-adjusted reference values for Finnish women and men. The formulas for the fitness index calculation are as follows:

Men:

420-(min x 11.6+ s x 0.20+ HR x 0.56+ BMI x 2.6)-agex0.2

Women:

304-(min x 8.5+ s x 0.14+ HR x 0.32+BMI x 1.1)-age x 0.4, where:

min= walking time, minutes

s= walking time, seconds

HR= heart rate at the finish, beats per minute

BMI= body mass index (body weight in kg divided by height in metres squared)

age= age in years

Equations for $\dot{V}O_2$max prediction (ml·min-1·kg-1) are as follows:

Men:

184.9-4.65 x time-0.22 x HR-0.26 x age-1.05 x BMI

Women:

116.2-2.98 x time-0.11 x HR-0.14 x age-0.39 x BMI, where

time= walking time in minutes.seconds, ie. 15min 30s = 15.50 min

HR=heart rate at the finish, beats per minute

BMI=Body mass index, kg·m2

age=age in years

Sources of error

The most common sources of error in the walking test are:

* Pretest prohibitions not complied with
* Inadequate warm-up and practice
* Too slow, too fast or uneven walking pace
* Delay in recording the postwalk heart rate
* Erroneous self-reported body weight

Evaluation of the results

The fitness index places individuals within a fitness category with respect to the persons of the same age (20-65 years-old) and sex:

<70   Markedly below average

70-89   Somewhat below average

90-110 Average

111-130 Somewhat above average

>130   Markedly above average

This classification is based on a Finnish population sample. The "avarage" category (90-110) covers one standard deviation around the mean, and the next categories up (111-130) and down (70-89) the further values within one standard deviation, or one half standard deviation each way. The extreme categories cover the remaining tail values.

When interpreting the results, it should be noted that a first test of an unaccustomed person may yield a slight underestimation of the true fitness, because of the unfamiliarity of fast walking.

NOTE: Detailed instructions for the organization, conduct and necessary calculations are given in "Guide for the UKK Institute 2-km walking test" (see Appendix 2).

Cycle ergometer test

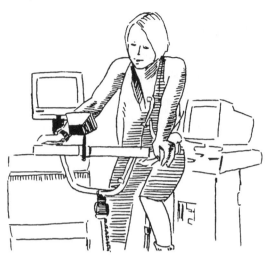

Aim

To estimate maximal aerobic power.

Background

Heart rate is generally recognized as the most useful variable as a basis of indirect tests of maximal aerobic power, because it displays a fairly linear response to increasing workloads and oxygen consumption. Heart rate normally reaches maximum value at or close to the same exercise intensity that produces maximal aerobic power. Predictive tests extrapolate $\dot{V}O_2max$ on the basis of one or more known heart rates at submaximal workloads and known (or estimated) maximum heart rate. Predictive tests assume also a constant oxygen consumption to power-output relationship throughout the test for all subjects.

This form of test is perhaps the most widely used method of assessing aerobic fitness. However a great variety of protocols exists. The common objective of all protocols is either to provide data to determine the work capacity at a certain heart rate (e.g. the PWC 170 protocol) or for the estimation of maximal oxygen uptake. The determination of physical work capacity at a standardised heart rate of 170 beats per minute is inappropriate for adults in middle age and beyond as maximum heart rate decreases with age. A satisfactory age related equivalent to 170 for young people (the notional ceiling of aerobic work) has not been established, although 85 % of maximum heart rate for age is sometimes used. The large variety of protocols arises because of different time constraints on conducting the test in different circumstances, and the different technical specifications of the available ergometres.

The criteria for satisfactory protocol are that the subject's heart rate should be brought via a series of progressive workloads to a value at the end of the final load of the order of 70-85 % maximal heart rate for age.

Description of the test

A simple protocol based on the description and guidelines for cycle ergometer testing endorsed by World Health Organization (Lange Andersen et al. 1971) and by The International Biological Programme, which has been used extensively is described below.

The subject pedals at three progressive workloads each for a period of 4 minutes preceded by a lighter warm up workload lasting 2 to 4 minutes. The final workload takes the subject to the order of 70-85 % of age-predicted maximum heart rate. The maximal oxygen uptake is then estimated from the relationship of heart rate to workload during the test assuming linearity.

Conditions for the test

• It is essential that the subject be in a calm and rested condition before embarking on the protocol and that adequate instruction is given in the nature of the test and the technique of pedalling.

• Vigilance over strict pedalling cadence is essential. 60 pedal revolutions per minute is recommended for the mechanically braked ergometer. If, however a constant power ergometer is available (which keeps the workload constant within a range of pedalling cadences) the subject may choose their own cadence to the extent of small variations around 60 revolutions and may be encouraged to pedal somewhat faster as the loads become heavier to avoid localised fatigue.

• The room should be well ventilated, preferably with a direct current of air (fan) playing on the subject and the environmental temperature somewhere between 15 and 25 degrees centigrade.

• Whatever ergometer is used, it is vital that it be accurately calibrated. Some ergometres, for example those with suspended weights in a cradle, are self calibrating. Others, particularly the electrically braked constant power variety, need frequent calibration checks and adjustment by a technically qualified person.

• Care should be taken that the subject has the saddle adjusted to the correct height, i.e. with the knee only slightly bent at the bottom of the down stroke, and that the handlebars are in a comfortable position.

Heart rate is recommended to be monitored throughout the exercise and should be measured with a reliable technique.

Equipment

* Manually or electrically braked cycle ergometer
* Heart rate recorder
* Clock
* Fan for ventilation
* Metronome (see note under "Problems")

Procedure

After adjustment to the saddle height and explanation of the test to the subject he/she begins pedalling and gradually builds up to the cadence of 60 pedal revolutions per minute. Loading at this stage is very light. This preliminary warm up load is used to give an indication of the condition of the subject and determines the subsequent initial workload proper. It also enables the subject to familiarize themselves with the exercise; usually the heart rate will subside and become more regular during this warm-up as the subject adjusts to the unfamiliar situation and the emotional component is suppressed.

Guidelines for suitable workloads are given in the table below. It must be emphasised that the loadings must be adjusted and the increments set according to the subject's continuing response throughout the test. For some individuals with very poor fitness the given initial workloads may be hard work and result in a too high heart rate level. In such cases even lighter workloads are to be used.

The heart rate is recorded at the end of each minute, except for the final minute of each stage where the heart rate is recorded some 15 to 20 seconds before the end of the minute in order to give time for a reappraisal of the next increment.

At the end of the final load the subject is asked to continue pedalling for a further 30 sec to 1 minute with the load reduced to the warm-up level and at a gradually reducing cadence. Vigilance of the subject's condition should continue throughout this phase.

Guidelines for workload (Watts) selection in the 3-stage (WHO) ergometer test

Physical activity	Young and middle-aged adults (20-50/55 years)				Older adults (50/55-60/65 years)			
	Warm-up	1	2	3	Warm-up	1	2	3
Physically very active	Women 100	125	150	175 W	50	75	100	125 W
	Men 100	150	200	250 W	50	100	150	175 W
Sedentary or physically moderately active	Women 50	75	100	125 W	25	50	75	100 W
	Men 50	100	150	175 W	50	75	100	125 W

The initial workload given in each series of four is for warming up (2-4 mins)

The targeted heart rate levels at each of the workloads proper (1, 2 & 3) should be of the following order:

<u>≤ 50 years-old</u>   <u>50 to 65 years-old</u>

Work load 1 110 - 120 beats/min   Work load 1 100 - 110 beats/min

Work load 2 130 - 140 beats/min   Work load 2 120 - 130 beats/min

Work load 3 145 - 165 beats/min   Work load 3 140 - 155 beats/min

<u>Calculations</u>

The estimation of maximal oxygen uptake is calculated from the heart rate responses to each of the 3 workloads proper (loads 1, 2 and 3) either by the equation below or by "line of best-fit" linear regression using the graphical format as in figure 1.

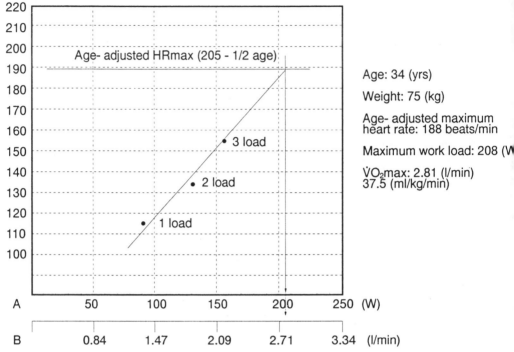

Heart rate
(beats/min)

Age- adjusted HRmax (205 - 1/2 age)

3 load

2 load

1 load

A

B

Age: 34 (yrs)

Weight: 75 (kg)

Age- adjusted maximum
heart rate: 188 beats/min

Maximum work load: 208 (W

$\dot{V}O_2$max: 2.81 (l/min)
37.5 (ml/kg/min)

**Figure 1: 12-minute cycle-test using the age adjusted maximal heart rate formula
derived from Finnish population.**

Three submaximal heart rates, maximum heart rate and three work loads are used for
estimation of maximum work output and $\dot{V}O_2$max.

$$Wmax\ (W) = 3.load(W) + \left[(HRmax - HR3) \times \frac{3.load(W) - \dfrac{1.load(W) + 2.load(W)}{2}}{HR3 - \dfrac{HR1\ +\ HR2}{2}} \right]$$

Where: Wmax = estimated maximal workload in watts

HR = heart rate at end of load

Example:

1. load 90 Watts HR1 115 beats/min

2. load 130 watts HR2 133 beats/min

3. load 160 Watts HR3 155 beats/min

HRmax 188 beats/min[1]

$$160 + \left[(188 - 155) \times \cfrac{160 - \cfrac{90 + 130}{2}}{155 - \cfrac{115 + 133}{2}} \right] = 208 \text{ Watts}$$

$$\dot{V}O_2\text{max (ml/kg/min)} = \frac{W\text{max(W)} \times 12.48 + 217}{\text{Body Weight (kg)}}$$

Example.

$$\frac{208 \times 12.48 + 217}{75} = 37.5 \text{ ml/kg/min}$$

Problems

Provided the conditions for testing and the criteria for a satisfactory protocol are complied with, few problems are likely to occur when cycle ergometry is administered by well-trained staff who can evaluate the subject's response and condition and adjust the increments accordingly. The most likely problems are however:

- The subject is not adequately calm or rested before the test
- Heart rate recording fails (make sure it works during early part of warm-up - stop and adjust if not).

1) NOTE. The extrapolation to estimated maximal heart rate uses a formula derived for the Finnish population tested (205-0.5 age in years, beats per minute). Other recent studies suggest that this more truly represents the age related decline than the steeper gradient represented by the traditional formula of 220-age. Ideally formulae should be derived for the population or its subsample being tested.

- The subject reaches target heart rate too early (experience in load setting will reduce this occurrence).

- The subject fails to reach a high enough heart rate in the final load (again experience will help to avoid this, but the solution may be an additional load in individual cases).

- Ergometer defective or out of calibration.

- The subject fails to maintain cadence (important only with mechanically loaded ergometer or electrical without constant power facility). A metronome to assist the tester in coaching the required cadence is often useful.

Evaluation of the results

Swedish population reference values in quintiles by age and sex are given in table 3, p. 95. These data were obtained from a submaximal cycle ergometer test with slightly different protocol from that described above, and calculated using the 220-age formula for maximum heart rate. For a full discussion of the evaluation of aerobic fitness test scores see Chapter 5.

Endurance shuttle run test

Aim

The 20 metre shuttle run test (20-MST) is a maximal test involving running which is performed indoors. The result is used as an index of cardiorespiratory endurance or to estimate maximal aerobic power ($\dot{V}O_2$max).

Background

Although not as universal as walking, running is a mode of exercise that can be performed by many adults. If performed for at least 5 to 6 minutes it reflects cardiovascular fitness. A widely used running test for assessing cardiovascular fitness is the 20-MST. The test was conceived to overcome the problems of pace-judgment inherent in most other walking/running tests.

Description of test

The test begins at a slow running pace (8 km/hour) and ends when the subject can no longer sustain the pace. Participants run a 20 metre piste, there and back continuously (one foot touching the end-line) in accordance with a pace dictated by a sound signal. The running speed is increased every minute by 0.5 km/hour, each minute constituting a stage (see table 1 to appendix 3). The subject should be required to stop if on 2 consecutive laps he/she fails to reach a line 3 m from the end of the piste or feels undue distress. The stage at which the subject drops out is the test result and serves as an indicator of his/her cardiorespiratory endurance. It is clear that the accuracy of the test depends on the strict application of the stop criteria. The length of the test varies according to the individual: the fitter the subject, the longer the test lasts.

Equipment needed for the test

* A gymnasium or space large enough to mark out a 20 metre piste
* A measuring tape
* Adhesive tape to mark the beginning and the end of the 20 metre piste
* A tape recorder, preferably with speed adjustment
* A pre-recorded tape containing the protocol (see Appendix 2)

Organization

The subjects should be informed prior to the test of the constraints regarding eating, exercise and stimulants. It is important to ensure that it is appropriate for the subject to perform a test of maximal aerobic power. The health questionnaire must be completed.When performing the test take the following into account:

- Study the graphic representation of the test protocol (see fig. 2).

- Select the test site; allow for a space of at least one metre at either end of the piste (ie. total length >22 m).

- The wider the area used, the greater the number of subjects that can be tested simultaneously: the space for each subject should be a minimum of one metre. If more than one subject is tested it is advisable to give each subject a clearly visible number.

- The surface should be uniform and non-slip but the material of which it is made is not important when the test is performed indoors. Shoes worn should grip well. The two ends of the 20 metre piste should be clearly marked.

- Check the functioning of the sound track and tape recorder. Ensure that the apparatus is powerful enough for everyone to hear.

- Listen to the contents of the sound track. Note the numbers on the tape position indicator so as to be able to locate the key sections of the tape quickly.

- Check the tape speed of the recorder or cassette player to be used on the day of the test. For this, use the one minute calibration period recorded at the beginning of the tape. If this calibration period differs by more than one second, adjust the turning speed of the tape recorder or alternatively adjust the running distance so that the subjects run at the correct speed (see Appendix 3, table 2). Note that a cassette-tape may stretch after having been used for several times.

The subject should stand on the start line and commence the test at the first 'BEEP'. They should be instructed to carefully follow the pace, and not run faster or slower than required.

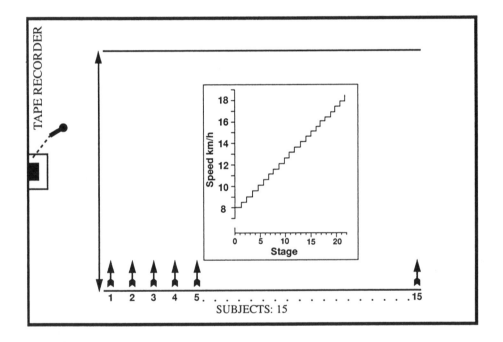

Figure 2: Graphic description of the endurance shuttle run test.

Scoring

After each subject stops, the last completed stage is noted with an accuracy of half a stage (see Appendix 3, table 1).

An alternative way of scoring is by counting each lap.

Calculations

The $\dot{V}O_2$max can be estimated from the test result by using a regression equation. Léger and Gadoury (1989) calculated a regression equation for the prediction of $\dot{V}O_2$max based on results of 53 males and 24 females ranging in age from 19 to 47 years. $\dot{V}O_2$max was measured directly during a maximal treadmill test. The following equation was found for both men and women:

$$\dot{V}O_2\text{max (ml/kg/min)} = -32.78 + 6.59x \quad (\text{x=maximal speed, r=0.90, SEE=4.4})$$

The limited number of subjects means that the application of these equations to the general public should be regarded as provisional.

Problems

This is a maximal test and requires scrupulous health screening. Therefore make sure that the health questionnaire is filled in and evaluated prior to the start of the test. When in doubt consult a medical doctor. This test may be unsuitable for people with orthopaedic problems. Unfit, older individuals may not be able to perform the test adequately (5-6 min) for a valid indication of aerobic fitness.

Evaluation of the results

One should realise the above mentioned limitation of the calculated $\dot{V}O_2$max values (e.g. derived from an equation that was calculated on the basis of small selected samples). The calculation of $\dot{V}O_2$max will give an error of about 4 ml/kg/min, as represented by the standard error of estimation (SEE). Therefore at the moment the best means of evaluating the test result of the endurance shuttle run is a 'within subject' comparison of the results achieved on two consecutive occasions.

Muscle strenght and endurance

Dynamic sit-up

Aim

Evaluation of trunk muscle strength and endurance.

Background

Trunk muscle strength is important for general movement, postural integrity and prevention of back and related problems. Conventional sit-up tests, such as the one in the Children's Eurofit battery (maximum number of sit-ups in 30 seconds) require maximal, and often exhausting effort and are potentially risky for older and/or unfit individuals. The presented modified three-stage test is purported to provide a safe test for all ages and, at the same time, to identify those individuals with functional inadequacy. Unfortunately the discriminatory power of the test is somewhat compromised as discussed later (p. 58).

Description of the test

The test is carried out in three sequential levels . The aim is to perform 5 repetitions of sit-ups on each level.

Conditions for the test

Subjects should be well informed about the procedure for the test, especially the position of the arms for the three levels and the starting and finishing position of each repetition.

Exclusion criteria

Dorsal and lumbar spine problems.

Procedure

The subject lies on his/her back with both knees bent at 90° . The tester holds the subject's feet. The first five sit-ups are done with the arms straight, palms resting on the thighs. The aim of each sit-up is to reach midpatella with the fingertips of both hands from a

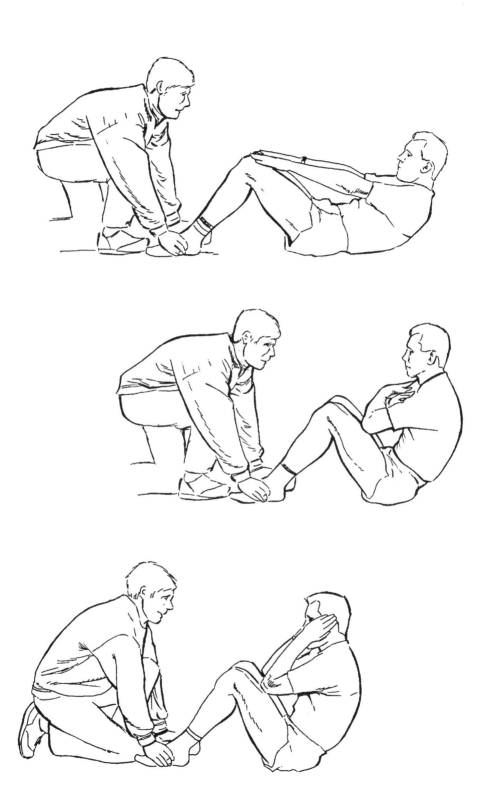

straight lying position. The next five sit-ups are done with the arms folded over the chest. The aim is to reach the thighs with both elbows. The last five sit-ups are performed with fingertips touching the back of the earlobes and again reaching the thighs with the elbows. Each of the five repetitions at each level should be done without pause. The interval between each level should be no longer than is necessary to teach the next movement.

Scoring

The number of completed repetitions is recorded (0-15).

Equipment

Gymnastic mat or soft carpet.

Problems

Subjects either do not return to the starting position between each repetition or fail to reach midpatella or thigh. Especially in stage 3 some subjects lose contact between fingers and the earlobes. Subject attempts to rest between the repetitions.

Evaluation of the results

Swedish population reference values in quintiles by age and sex are given in table 4, p.96. As seen in the table, the test does not discriminate the relative fitness over the whole age distribution, but rather identifies low fitness in individuals over the age of 30-35 years. If a discriminatory test for younger and/or fitter individuals is required, a maximal sit-up test, such as number of sit-ups in 30 seconds (see Children's Eurofit) could be used.

There are no precise health-related criterion norms. In the Swedish study (Engström et al. 1993) a cut-off point of 5 repetitions was chosen as an arbitrary indication of poor trunk muscle function.

Flexibility Tests

Poor flexibility in selected joints may cause musculo-skeletal problems, especially around the shoulder, lumbar and hip regions. Stretching and flexibility exercises are known to reduce the incidence of these problems. It is not possible to measure general flexibility by one test such as the sit and reach test, which only evaluates the flexibility of the back and full stretch length of the hamstring muscles. It is important to notice that extreme flexibility is not a goal for health-related fitness, but may in fact be harmful in some cases.

Side-bending of the trunk

Aim

To measure the extent of lateral flexion of the thoracic and lumbar spine.

Background

Subjects with back pain or poor function often present limitations in spinal flexibility. Measures of lateral flexion have been shown to correlate with indices of back health.

Description of the test

The aim is to bend laterally first to the subject's right and then to his/her left as far as possible from the upright standing position .

Conditions for the test

The position of the feet must be standardized as described below. No rotation of the trunk or movement of the pelvic area is allowed; both heels must stay in contact with the floor. The subject wears shorts.

Procedure

The subject stands upright against a wall on two parallel lines at right angles to the wall and 15 cm apart. The scapulae and buttocks are in contact with the wall and the heels slightly away from the wall so that a comfortable upright stance can be maintained. Arms are held straight against the sides of the body. The position of the middle finger on each side is marked with a horizontal line on the lateral thigh. The subject is then asked to bend sideways as far as possible while maintaining contact between back and wall. During the movement the middle finger is slid down along the thigh. The end position, which is held for 1-2 seconds is then marked on the thigh. The distance between the markings on each thigh is then measured.

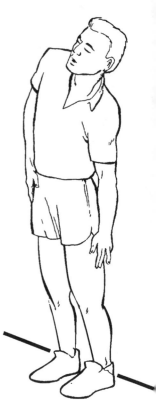

Scoring

The test score is the distance the finger tips move down the leg during maximum lateral bending. The results are recorded for both sides, added together and divided by two to produce an average side-bending score. The difference between right and left sides can be used as an additional index.

Equipment
* cloth tape measure
* marker pen

Problems
Subjects rotate their trunk or move their pelvis sideways while bending.

Evaluation of the results
There are no health-related criteria available for the side-bending test. Therefore population norm values should be used for the evaluation of the results. Persons with poor values may benefit from exercises that improve trunk mobility. Also extreme hypermobility deserves attention, since it may be indicative of increased risk for back problems. In such cases stabilization of the spine via the strengthening of the back muscles may be beneficial.

Finnish reference values in quintiles by age and sex are given in table 5, p. 97.

Sit-and-reach

<u>Aim</u>

Evaluation of trunk flexibility and hamstring 'tightness'.

<u>Background</u>

The sit-and-reach test is included in the battery largely because of its almost universal usage in existing test batteries, and a consensus of opinion that poor scores are associated with back problems. Recent evidence to support this opinion is however controversial as is the validity of the measure with regard to flexibility of the trunk.

<u>Description of test</u>

The subject sits on the floor with straight legs and reaches as far as possible forward.

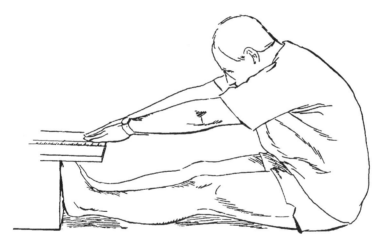

<u>Conditions for the test</u>

Standardized warm-up procedure is necessary for the proper and safe administration of the test. For this purpose a preliminary trial of the movement should be performed without maximal effort. The test should be carried out without shoes.

<u>Exclusion criteria</u>

Problems of the lumbar spine. If subjects experience back pain or discomfort during the test, it should be discontinued.

Procedure

The procedure begins by the tester demonstrating the manoeuvre. The subject is then asked to do a practice movement followed by two maximal efforts. For the three performances the tester stands beside the subject with hands on the knees of the subject to ensure that the legs are kept straight. The subject bends slowly forward, trying to reach as far as possible along the scale on the box pushing the ruler with extended fingertips. The subject should hold the final position steady for 2-3 seconds without bouncing.

Scoring

The two maximal trials are measured to the nearest centimetre read from the scale. Thus, reaching to the level of the vertical edge supporting the feet will score 25; reaching a further 7 cm will score 32. The better score is recorded.

Note!

Some sit-and-reach boxes, otherwise having the same dimensions as described below, use a different measurement scale in which for instance a score of 15 cm, as in the Children's Eurofit box, equals the level of the vertical edge supporting the feet. As adults as a group have poorer flexibility than children, longer extention of the top plate is necessary.

Some sit and reach boxes have both a dimension and a measurement scale that differs from the standard described.

Obviously different dimensions and different measurement scales have implications for the interpretation of test results. Therefor one should check the dimensions of the sit and reach box and the measurement scale before using it.

Equipment

A test table or box 32 cm in height and 50 cm long, has a top plate 45 cm wide. The length of the top plate is 75 cm, the first 25 cm of which extend over the front edge of the box towards the subject (the soles of the subject's feet are placed against the front end of the box). The measurement scale extends the full length of the top plate reading from 0 to 75 cm. A ruler about 30 cm long is placed across the scale for the subject to push forward with the fingertips. For a commercial box see Appendix 2.

Bent knees and/or bouncing towards the end of the effort.

Swedish reference values in quintiles by age and sex are given in table 6, p.98. No health-related criterion values are available (see discussion in Chapter 5).

Motor fitness

Single leg balance test

Aim

Evaluating whole body balance.

Background

Balance contributes to general physical performance but also to the prevention of injuries, especially in the elderly (see Chapter 4).

Description of test

General balance is evaluated as the ability to balance on one leg on a flat firm surface with the eyes closed . The number of attempts to achieve a total duration of 30 seconds in balance is measured.

Conditions for the test

The test is performed in bare or stockinged feet. The preferred leg is used (same leg throughout the test). Two short pretrials are performed. Movement of the arms and the free leg is allowed. Hopping or shifting the position of the supporting foot is not allowed.

Exclusion criteria

Arthritic conditions or pain in lower limb joints.

CHAPTER 6

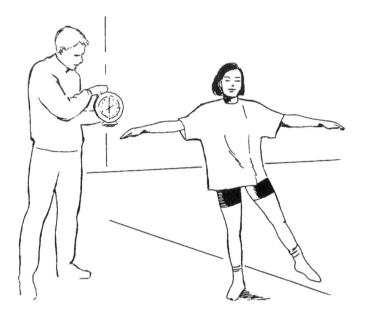

Procedure

The clock is started as soon as the subject achieves balance. If the subject loses balance, the clock is stopped and the subject tries again immediately.

Scoring

Number of attempts in total accumulated time of 30 seconds. If the subject loses his or her balance 15 times within the first total of 15 seconds or is unable to stand on one leg, the test result is 30.

Problems

Some individuals have problems with having the eyes closed for 30 seconds. In fact some subjects can not keep balance at all with the eyes closed, and thus, they do not close their eyes completely. Furthermore, he or she may touch the floor with their free foot. This should be regarded as a failure and the score increased by one, although the clock is not stopped.

Equipment needed

* A stop watch.
* Open, firm floor area

Evaluation of the results

Swedish population norms in quintiles by age and sex are given in table 7,p. 99. There are no criterion values available (see discussion in Chapter 5).

2nd priority tests

Musculoskeletal fitness

Vertical jump

Aim

To measure maximal vertical jump ability, which reflects maximal leg muscle strength, power and coordination.

Background

Leg muscle strength is a vital factor for general activity and functional health. It becomes especially critical with advancing age. It can only be measured directly with laboratory facilities. Therefore, the vertical jump provides a simple field test for evaluating this physiological factor.

Description of test

The height of the vertical jump is measured using a measuring-tape, one end attached to a belt placed around the waist and the other free end sliding under a plate on the floor .

Conditions for the test

The subject must be well informed about the procedure for the test. A general warm-up period of some minutes and one or two pretrials are needed. Sports shoes should be used.

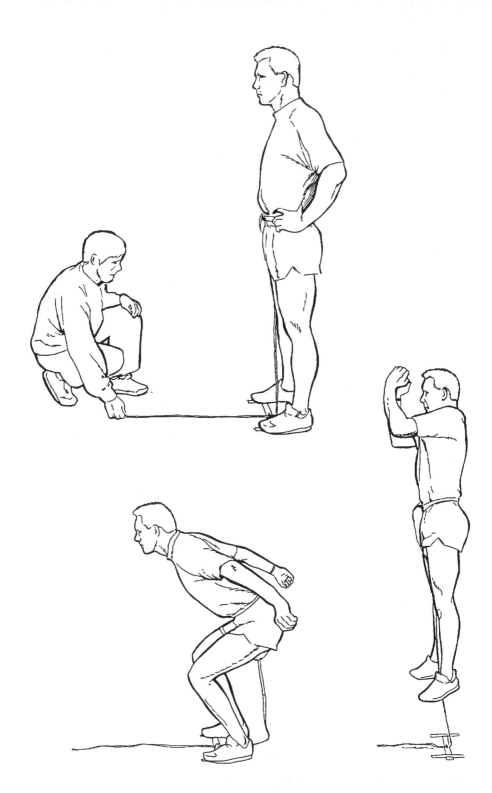

Symptoms of spine and lower extremities, severe obesity.

Procedure

The subject stands with the legs straight and somewhat apart over the plate. The tester records the number on the measuring-tape at the plate. The subject jumps vertically as high as possible using a rhythmic counter movement and arm swing to aid the jump. The subject must land within a few centimetres of the take-off point.

Scoring

The height of the vertical jump is measured in centimetres. The best result of 2-3 trials is used.

Equipment

* A measuring-tape attached to a belt, which has a buckle for adjustment of different waistgirth.
* A measuring plate mounted on the floor.

Evaluation of the results

Swedish population norms in quintiles by age and sex are given in table 8, p. 100. No health-related criterion norms are currently available (see discussion in Chapter 5). In the interpretation of the test results it is to be noted that excess weight reduces the jumping performance and thus the score is a measure of relative rather than absolute muscle power.

Bent arm hang

Aim

To test static muscular endurance of arms and shoulders.

Background

This test is similar to the bent arm hang test in the Children's Eurofit except that an undergrasp grip is used. This makes the test easier and allows more adults to achieve a measurable performance. While many adults could perform the more difficult version, such people will also perform relatively better with the easier version. In choosing this test the over-riding consideration was to provide the same test for all adults.

Description of test

The test task is to hold the arms bent as long as possible while hanging free from a bar with the hands in undergrasp position. The height of the bar should be adjusted to accommodate the tallest subjects.

Conditions for the test

Subjects should be well informed about the test procedure. The test is performed in stockinged or bare feet. Only one trial without practice is performed.

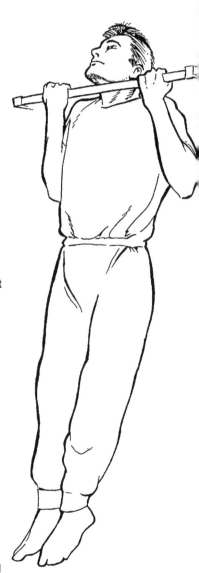

Procedure

The subject takes up position under the bar, grips it undergrasp, that is with the palms of hands facing him or her and the thumbs round, at about shoulder width. The tester helps lift the subject until the chin is just above the level of the bar. The position is held for as long as possible. The subject must not rest his or her chin on the bar. The test ends when the eyes are below the level of the bar.

The stopwatch is started at the moment where the subject unaided has his or her chin at the or above level of the bar. The subject should be stopped from swinging, and encouraged during the test. The bar is cleaned with a cloth before each subject. Chalk on the hands will improve grip. With the smaller subjects a bench or chair can be used to achieve the initial position.

Scoring

This is scored in tenths of a second, e.g. a time of 17.4 seconds is a score of 174. A time of 1 minute 3 seconds and 5 tenths is a score of 6035.

* A metal bar of 2.5 cm in diametre (eg. a gymnastic horizontal bar) placed horizontally above the ground so that the subject can reach and grip it without jumping.
* A stopwatch.
* A soft mat placed beneath the bar.
* Magnesium chalk.
* Cloth.
* A bench or chair.

Problems

Subject expends significant energy achieving the start position. Use height adjustment and/or bench to minimise this.

Subject allowed to swing or sway.

Evaluation of the results

There are no population norms nor health-related criterion norms currently available for adults.

Flexibility

Shoulder abduction

Aim

To measure the shoulder abduction range of motion on the dominant or preferred side.

Background

Shoulder abduction is the movement involved in reaching for objects above head level or at the back of the neck. Restriction in shoulder joint range of motion limits activities of daily living especially in the elderly.

Description of the test

The subject is seated with the lumbar spine against a vertical guide, and the arm to be measured hanging vertically at the side. The arm is raised through a plane of movement 45° to the frontal plane to achieve the maximum elevated position.

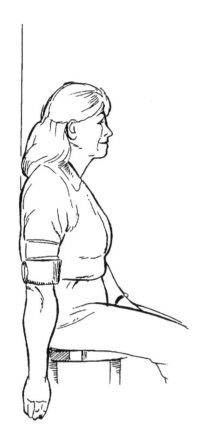

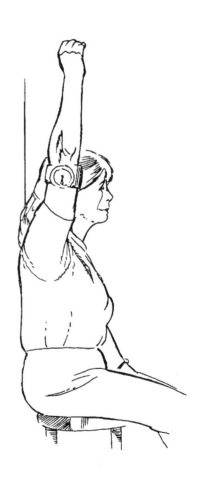

Conditions for the test

The subject removes outer clothing. The measured arm is bared.

Exclusion criteria

Subjects who have a recent history of shoulder dislocation or related surgery should be excluded from this test. If the problem applies to one side only, the opposite shoulder can be measured.

Procedure

The range of movement is measured as the maximal number of degrees of arc through which the arm moves upwards in 45° horizontal flexion, from hanging vertically by the side, thumb forwards. The measurement is explained briefly to the subject. Sleeves are pushed to the top of the arm. The goniometre strap is attached to the upper arm at the mid-point between the acromial and olecranon processes. The goniometre is attached to the strap facing directly backwards. The shoulder abduction manoeuvre is then described and demonstrated to the subject.

The subject is then seated, with the centre of the back against a vertical guide such as the leading edge of an opened door. The subject looks straight ahead keeping the shoulders horizontal and maintaining contact with the vertical guide at the level of the lumbar spine. With the arm hanging freely at the side of the body, the goniometre is set at zero. The subject is instructed to swing his or her arm slowly up towards the head and back as far as possible so that the hand travels in an arc midway between the forwards and sideways position. The position is held at the limit of the movement until the measurement is made. The angular range achieved is read directly from the goniometre dial and recorded to the nearest 2°.

If the dominant side is injured, the measurement is made on the other side, this fact being recorded. The subject should carry out all manoeuvres in a smooth controlled manner. The administrator must check that the subject's arm is hanging freely at the side and that the plane of movement is at 45°. The lumbar contact must not be lost.

The measurement is repeated, including checking and resetting 0, until two measures within 5° of one another have been obtained. Three measures are standard unless the third score exceeds the previous better score by more than 5°, in which case a further measure is made up to a maximum of 5 measures.

Scoring

The best score of the 2 or more scores within the defined limits of agreement (5°) is recorded.

Equipment

* A gravity goniometre (see Appendix 2) attached to a strap to accommodate differing upper arm girths.

* A vertical guide projecting from the wall with a light operating contact switch helps to ensure the correct back position.

* A stool of approximately 50 cm in height.

Problems

It is important to check that the shoulders are level throughout the movement. The goniometre dial must be firmly tapped before reading to ensure that the indicator is not stuck against the dial.

Evaluation of the results

English reference values in quintiles by age and sex are given in table 9, p. 101.

Preliminary studies among older people have shown a range of movement of less than 120° to be functionally restrictive for many daily tasks. Leisure and sports activities will often impose higher thresholds. As an age-related decline is normal, particularly among post-menopausal women, greater ranges of movement need to be maintained in younger adults, so that such decline does not reach disabling levels with ageing.

Musculoskeletal fitness

Hand grip

Aim

To measure static grip strength.

Background

Sufficient grip strength is required for performing many everyday functions and tasks such as opening cans and bottles, pulling plugs from sockets and holding on to handrails. It also reflects more general muscle strength.

Description of test

Handgrip strength is measured with a hand dynamometre . The task is to squeeze the dynamometre as forcefully as possible. The test is carried out twice with the dynamometre held in the preferred hand.

Conditions for the test

The tester describes and demonstrates the test and the subject is asked to do one pretrial in order to secure a comfortable grip on the dynamometre. No extraneous movements such as jerking of the arm or body are allowed.

Exclusion criteria

Subjects with high blood pressure should not perform the test without consulting their physician. The test is not suitable for persons with joint problems of the test arm.

Procedure

The subject stands in an upright position with the dynamometre in the preferred hand, slightly away from the body, with the scale facing the tester. The arm should be straight.

The grip of the dynamometre should be adjusted to the size of the hand to bring the second joint of the fore-finger approximately to a right angle. This is usually consistent with subjective impression of the optimal grip size. The dynamometre should be squeezed firmly and gradually, building quickly up to maximum force. The test is performed twice, with an interval of about 10 seconds between trials.

Scoring

The better result of the two attempts is the score. It is recorded in kilograms (to the nearest kg). Since muscle strength and its sufficiency in many situations is related to body weight, the test result may also be usefully expressed relative to body weight (ie. kg/kg body weight).

Equipment

A calibrated hand dynamometre with adjustable grip (see Appendix 2).

Problems

The test does not give optimal results if the grip size of the dynamometre is not adjusted to the size of the hand, particularly if the subject's hands are very large or small.

Subjects with sweaty hands may experience difficulties in performing the test. A cloth should be provided.

Evaluation

English population norms in quintiles by age and sex are given in table 10, p. 102. No health-related criteria are available (see discussion in Chapter 5).

Plate tapping

Aim

To measure the speed of repeated limb movement during a defined, semi-precise task.

Background

Coordination and speed of limb movement are components of manual dexterity, which are needed in most everyday manual tasks.

Description of test

Speed of limb movement is measured with the help of a plate tapping table, adjustable in height. The aim of the test is touch two discs alternately with the preferred hand as fast as possible, completing 25 full cycles.

Conditions for the test

The subject must be well informed about the procedure for the test. A general warm-up is allowed. The test is not suitable for persons with joint problems of the hand, elbow or shoulder.

Procedure

The subject stands at the plate tapping table, with the non-preferred hand on the rectangular plate in the centre of the table. The preferred hand is placed on the opposite disc so that the hands are crossed. The preferred hand is then moved back and forth between the two discs, as quickly as possible (for 25 full cycles ie. there and back) over the hand in the middle. The test is performed twice, with a short rest interval in between. The subject is allowed to have a short trial before the test in order to select the preferred hand.

The tester should make sure that:

- the height of the table is adjusted to the size of the subject, such that the edge of the table is just below the waist level
- the stopwatch used for timing the 25 cycles is started at the signal "ready...start!"
- the subject keeps one hand on the rectangular plate during the whole test.

Scoring

The better result of two attempts recorded in tenths of a second is the score.

If a subject fails to touch a disc, an extra cycle is added in order to reach the required 25 full cycles.

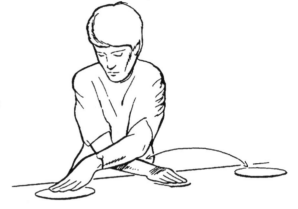

Equipment

* A table adjustable in height.
* Two rubber discs, each 20 centimetres in diametre, are fixed to the table. The centre points of the discs are 80 centimetres apart.
* A rectangular plate (10 x 20 centimetres) is placed half way between the two discs.
* A stopwatch.

Problems

Subjects sometimes tend to slide the hands over each other, or let the hands touch each other. This should not be allowed. At first the subject can be warned, but if this occurs more than a couple of times the test has to be stopped and started all over again.

Evaluation of the results

No population norms or health-related criteria are available for adult populations (see discussion in Chapter 5).

Skinfolds

Background

In recent years, the concept of fat percentage and the assumptions upon which the most common existing methods to measure fat rely, have been widely discussed. In terms of feasibility, the measurement of skinfold thickness, when trained evaluators follow standardized techniques, remains one of the easiest and most accessible means of assessing subcutaneous fat in the field setting. A skinfold includes a double layer of skin, of varying width, depending on the site, and the underlying adipose tissue. While new methods have been developed to estimate fat percentages eg. near-infrared interactance, and bioelectric impedance, these are also indirect methods and skinfolds remain the field technique of choice.

In studies that include skinfold measurements, the raw values of the caliper readings are usually converted to fat percentage by means of one or more validated equations. These equations are population specific, and are not valid for subjects of different ethnicity. For this reason, there is an increasing tendency to describe the values in millimetres of the individual skinfolds, or the sum of them. Moreover, the monitoring of skinfold measurements by reliable evaluators, provides information about individual variations and changes in subcutaneous fat distribution.

CHAPTER 6

General technique for obtaining skinfolds

1. All measures should be made on the right side of the body.

2. The skinfold site is located and marked on the skin.

3. The thumb and index finger of the left hand are placed on the skin wide enough apart to ensure inclusion of the fat layer, and the skinfold is picked up just above (1 cm) or laterally (1 cm) to the mark previously mentioned for vertical or horizontal folds

respectively. The skinfold is raised by a pinching, slightly rolling action. The amount of skin elevated must form a fold with approximately parallel sides, and should be grasped firmly throughout the measurement.

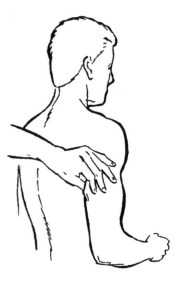

4. The calipers are applied to the middle of the elevated fold, with the near edge of the pressure plate of the calipers about 1 cm from the grasping fingers and thumb.

5. Relative stabilization of the reading occurs at about two seconds. The reading should be recorded at this point. The calipers should be kept at right angles to the fold and not twisted.

6. An average is taken of two readings that should not differ by more than five per cent. If the difference is greater, a third reading should be taken and the average of the two closer readings recorded.

Equipment
 * Harpenden type calipers (see Appendix 2).
 * Skin pencil.

Measurement sites
Four sites - biceps, triceps, subscapular, and suprailic are recommended, allowing the use the prediction equations for percentage body fat proposed by Durnin and Womersley (1974) as shown in table 11, p. 103.

Biceps skinfold

The subject stands, with the arm held relaxed at his or her side. A point is located halfway between the acromial process and the olecranon, and marked on the skin. The skinfold is picked up over the belly of the biceps at the marked site on a vertical line joining the centre of the antecubital fossa to the head of the humerus.

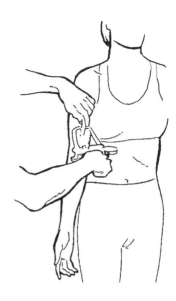

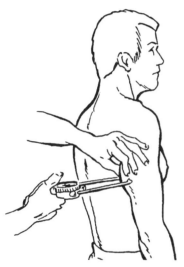

Triceps skinfold

The subject stands, with arm relaxed and the palm of the hand facing forwards. The skinfold is picked up over the surface of the triceps muscle just above the previously marked site, on a vertical line from the olecranon to the acromion.

Subscapular skinfold

The subject stands as for the triceps skinfold, with the shoulders and arms relaxed. The medial (vertebral) border of the scapula is palpated and the inferior angle located. The skinfold is picked up immediately below the inferior angle of the scapula with the fold running on a diagonal approximately 45° to the horizontal (obliquely downwards and outwards).

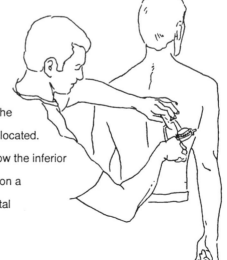

Suprailiac skinfold

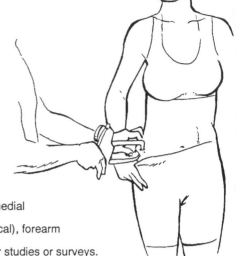

The subject stands, with his or her right arm slightly abducted so as to give easy access the measuring site. A horizontal fold is located immediately above the iliac crest on the midaxillary line.

Other commonly used skinfolds eg: front thigh, medial calf, pectoral (chest), midaxillary, abdominal (umbilical), forearm etc. may be selected for comparisons with particular studies or surveys.

Weight

Beam scales or accurate electronic scales should be used to measure weight (see Appendix 2). Spring scales are not recommended for this purpose.

The subject, wearing minimal clothing, stands straight and still over the center of the scale platform, with body weight evenly distributed between both feet. Weight is recorded to the nearest tenth of kilogram, and the time of the day at which measurements are made should also be recorded, as diurnal variations of about 2 kg are seen in adults.

Height

Ideally stature should be recorded with a stadiometre (see Appendix 2). If this is not the case an anthropometre or wall-scale - with an accuracy required of at least ± 1 cm - can be used. Whenever possible an assistant aids the evaluator in obtaining this measurement.

Footwear should be removed and hair should be compressed on top of the scalp by the measuring device.

Body Mass Index

This index of relative weight, also known as Quetelet's Index is calculated as body weight in kg divided by the square of the height in metres (kg/m^2).

Waist to hip ratio

The ratio of the waist circumference to the hip circumference reflects intra-abdominal fatness, and a high ratio is considered to be a cardiovascular risk indicator.

Waist circumference

The subject stands erect and relaxed, arms at the sides and feet together. The measurement is taken at the mid-point between the costal margin and iliac crest at the mid-axillary line using a non-stretch tape in a horizontal plane. With the subject breathing gently the mid-point between inhalation and exhalation is measured.

Hip (buttocks or gluteal) circumference

The subject wears minimal clothing (eg. swimsuit or underwear), and stands erect, with the feet together, and arms slightly forward in order to facilitate the positioning of the tape. The tester - at one side of the subject - places the tape around the buttocks in a horizontal plane at the level of the greater trochanters. The tape is moved downwards from this position and the greatest girth recorded.

Evaluation of anthropometry

BMI is the most frequently used clinical measure for determining relative fatness, despite the fact that as a measure of relative weight, it cannot reliably indicate the preponderance of fat rather than muscle. Commonly doctors and health educators will use the following categories.

BMI =   less than 20 - underweight

          20-25 -acceptable

          greater than 25 but less than 30 - overweight

          greater than 30 - obese

          greater than 40 - severely obese

Whereas these categories are useful guidelines in monitoring the direction of change in relative weight, and are for most individuals appropriate with regard to the obesity category, in that a BMI in excess of 30 is associated with health risk, there are some dangers in their use. "Underweight" and "overweight", particularly when labelling categories either side of 'acceptable', are terms which imply health risk, whereas reviews of the health risk of obesity and overweight do not entirely support that implication. Thus Pi-Sunyer (1991) found no significant health risk associated with BMI from 25-27 (about 1/5 of the English population). Some authorities extend this further, claiming that little or no health risk exists until BMI exceeds the order of 28 for men and 29 for women. Some studies even indicate that somewhat higher than average relative weight may be advantageous to health status and expectation in older people. A recent longitudinal study of American women (Willet et al. 1995) does however identify increased risk of CHD associated with increasing BMI within the so-called 'acceptable' relative weight range. It should be appreciated that for any given individual family history and other factors which predispose to coronary heart disease on the one hand or to cancers and respiratory disease on the other, should be taken into account when assessing the health risk associated with their relative weight.

Counselling individuals must be undertaken with caution as the consequence of inappropriate advice may be considerable unnecessary stress for the individual concerned, and at worst, the encouragement of truly health-threatening weight loss or 'weight cycling', especially among women.

A reasonable sequential evaluation of health threatening overweight would seem to be as follows:

(1)   high BMI = possible health risk
(2)   high BMI + high percentage body fat = probable health risk
(3)   high BMI + high body fat percentage + high waist/hip ratio = very probable health
       risk

The conventional thresholds of 25 and 30 for BMI signifying "overweight" and "obesity" can be adopted in this 3 stage appraisal, although values between 25 and 27 should not necessarily be interpreted as justifying the need for weight reduction unless body fat and/or waist to hip ratio are also above criterion values.

Estimated body fat percentage increases with age for a given value of relative weight. Thus the mean % body fat at the conventional BMI thresholds of 20, 25 and 30 increases in both sexes with age up to age 65 in the English population (see table 12, p. 104).

A reasonable guideline for health-threatening excess body fat might be of the order of 3-5 % above the mean % body fat for a given age and sex at a BMI more than 25. Thus, for example, a woman aged 40 whose BMI was 26 and who had more than 38 % body fat would appear to have a health need for weight reduction via fat loss. This would be consolidated if her waist measurement were more than 80 % of her hip girth.

The waist to hip ratio thresholds for increased cardiovascular disease risk are 1.00 for men (ie. waist girth equals or exceeds hip girth) and 0.8 for women, according to Larsson et al. (1984).

Of these three separate but associated criteria for overweight, distribution of fat, ie. abdominally, appears increasingly to be the most important in predicting cardiovascular disease.

The health risks of underweight, and the negative effect on psychological welfare and physical health of obsessive preoccupation with weight loss should always be borne in mind. Ideally, advice should emphasise the positive benefits of exercise as opposed to restrictive diet, and play down the importance of weight loss as an objective in itself. Rapid, substantial weight changes in either direction appear to be undesirable.

CHAPTER 6

CHAPTER 7

ASSESSMENT OF PHYSICAL ACTIVITY
AND HEALTH STATUS

Assessment of physical activity

<u>Why assess Physical Activity?</u>

Despite its lack of precision, information about people's physical activity and other aspects of their lifestyle, such as smoking behaviour and nutrition, is invaluable. The type of information which is useful depends on the nature of the investigation. This may range from the assembling of as much information as possible about a given individual in order to give them the best advice and prescription with regard to exercise, to a full-scale descriptive survey of a large population with an epidemiological dimension. In the latter case, the whole pattern and inter-relationship of all the physical measures and determinants of physical activity behaviour can be analyzed over time alongside data on morbidity and mortality, towards a better understanding of the relationship between physical activity, fitness and health.

<u>What determines physical activity behaviour?</u>

Physical activity is a form of human behaviour, and when trying to understand or counsel health-related behaviour it is useful to be aware of its determinants. A questionnaire about physical activity will be most useful if it also probes the nature of these determinants - the 'why' and 'why not' of participation.

In general three factors are distinguished as determinants of health-related behaviour: (a) attitude (b) social influence and (c) 'self-efficacy-cum-barriers' (Kok & Bouter 1990). Attitude refers to the knowledge and beliefs of a person concerning the specific consequences of a certain behaviour. An example of a positive attitude is: 'I want to participate in an employee fitness class because it is good for my health'. An example of a negative attitude is: 'I don't want to participate in an employee fitness class because it makes me sweat which is not practical since I have to work for another two hours'. It is the weighing process between the positive and the negative attitude that makes up the 'final' attitude. In this weighing process health is only seen as one of the considerations and is often an unimportant one.

Social influence is the influence by others; directly by what others expect, indirectly by what others do (modelling). An example of direct social influence is 'the positive expectation of my boss regarding my participation in an employee fitness class'. An example of indirect social influence is 'the fact that all my colleagues actively participate in an employee fitness class'. Social influence is often underestimated as a determinant of behaviour. It can lead to behaviour that conflicts with above mentioned attitudes. Most sports and physical activity situations are social situations.

'Self-efficacy-cum-barriers' stands for the determinant whether one is able to perform the (desired) behaviour. Self-efficacy is the person's perception of the ability to perform the behaviour, and barriers are the real problems people face in actually performing the behaviour. This determinant involves an estimation of ability (e.g. 'can I really do all these exercises at the employee fitness class?') taking into account possible internal (e.g. 'do I have sufficient skills, knowledge, endurance, etc. to actually perform the exercise?') or external barriers (e.g. 'do I have enough time to participate?' or 'do I have enough money to pay for the class and the sports clothing?').

These determinants are clearly inter-related. When trying to assess or modify physical activity behaviour it is important to be aware of these determinants and their influence on the individual or population concerned.

<u>Fitness assesment as a tool for individual counselling</u>
Increasingly sedentary people of all ages are being persuaded to take more exercise for the sake of their health. Often these individuals will arrive at a leisure centre and expect to have a fitness test and consultation, with a view to undertaking some form of prescribed exercise regimen or activities. In some countries referral schemes are in operation whereby physicians may send patients to nearby leisure centres for such a prescription.

If exercise is to become a sustained component of the person's lifestyle, then it has to be appropriate and fulfilling for the individual in its own right, which usually means that it must also be enjoyed. As well as poor fitness, the individual may have many other barriers to further participation, as explained above, as well as various attitudes and misconceptions about the demands and consequences of exertion. He or she will have sometimes straightforward, sometimes very complex and covert reasons for taking exercise, and expectations may be inconsistent with health needs or achievable goals.

While an informal, friendly atmosphere is essential to obtain the best quality of such information, a structured approach will ensure that nothing important is omitted. It will also ensure that the information can be recorded in a way which enables comparison, either with other individuals where appropriate, or more usually on subsequent occasions with the same individual. Whereas detailed qualitative information is needed, it is still useful to have a system whereby key features can be quantified or categorised. For example a numerical index might be given for 'total current physical activity' and a category for 'perceived barriers to exertion'.

In a counselling situation it is useful to find out what activity the person may have enjoyed in the past, what their reasons were for discontinuing and what activities might appeal that they haven't yet attempted. The person's access to available physical activity in terms of both time and place are also important pieces of information, as may be their preference for exercising with other people or on their own and in a competitive or non-competitive situation. Family status is also relevant as are the attitudes and activities of friends, relatives and colleagues. Together with this it is desirable to collect information regarding medical or physical constraints on exercise which might not be revealed by the fitness testing or the preliminary screening.

Many suitable interview-type questionnaire formats have been devised for counselling purposes but each for a specific population or set of circumstances. It is likely that this will always be the necessary approach, as a generalised questionnaire to suit all situations in all the member states is difficult to conceive and likely to be less acceptable than one which is purpose-designed.

CHAPTER 7

Questionnaire Design for Survey and
Epidemiological Use alongside Fitness Measures

The amount of information collected in this sort of approach is dependent on the resources of the investigation. These include time and what is an appropriate respondent burden. The information collected should be as objective as possible and convertible to data in digital form. The process whereby the subject's not always clear and precise response is converted to a numerical value must be credible. It is generally agreed that better information is obtained from questionnaires conducted via an interview than by self completion. This is only the case if the approach of the interviewers is consistent. In a large scale descriptive survey such as a national fitness and physical activity survey, where it may be appropriate to conduct a fairly lengthy interview questionnaire, a great deal of detail may be obtainable. It would, however, appear sensible to go for detail which one can envisage being able to analyze and which will be of use. However, there are also dangers in designing an investigation of this type in terms only of expected outcomes.

What type of information?

In designing a questionnaire for research purposes one should first determine what type of information is needed. The principal objective of a questionnaire used in a population survey of health, fitness and physical activity is to assess the type, nature, intensity and frequency of physical activity for each individual. This may comprise an inventory of all **current**, **recent**, **past** and ideally, **lifetime physical activity**. This can result in a very large amount of information which may require daunting resources for analysis with uncertain return. Many attempts have been made to arrive at a small number of relatively simple questions which provide the essence of the required information. Such questions may be just as useful as the more complex approach in providing indices of, for example, total physical activity or type of physical activity, but do not lend themselves to providing information for detailed strategy on the promotion of exercise.

Most survey questionnaires attempt to assemble information on physical activity in **occupation**, in **leisure**, and incidental to **everyday life**, e.g. walking and climbing stairs. Some questionnaires also include questions which seek to assess a person's **disposition towards exertion**, for example whether they tend to 'run for a bus' or 'run up flights of stairs', indeed their physical 'busyness'. This kind of information regarding lifestyle physical activity behaviour is the most difficult to quantify, for obvious reasons.

However, the assessment of this component is of great importance since for many people it is the most frequent, if not the only, feature of exercise in their everyday lives.

Some of the earliest major epidemiological studies which identified physical activity as being important to cardiovascular health were concerned with occupational physical activity and walking to work. Since these early studies, both such activities have declined dramatically. Hence it has been assumed, with some justification, that the variable "exercise" is principally defined by physical activity in leisure time. While this is largely true, the use of muscles to get about i.e. **walking** and **cycling** as a means of personal transport, constitutes for many individuals a much more regular and consistent exercise habit than a specified active leisure pursuit. For this reason it is important that a questionnaire should include effective questions quantifying this activity.

Level of intensity and energy expenditure.

One of the problems which beset the assessment of physical activity of individuals is the difficulty of attributing a **level of intensity** to the reported activity. This is further complicated by the fact that intensity can be either **absolute**, in terms of a fixed rate of energy expenditure for a given task or sport, e.g. playing squash is a very vigorous activity requiring an energy expenditure of 12 or more times resting level, or **relative** to the individual concerned, e.g. "playing club badminton makes me sweat and breathe hard".

Absolute levels of intensity of activities can be classified according to Ainsworth et al. (1993) by assigning an intensity unit to a certain activity. The applied intensity unit is the 'MET'. The MET value is defined as the ratio between the metabolic rate associated with the specified activity divided by the resting metabolic rate. One MET is also defined as the energy expenditure for sitting quietly, which is for the average individual approximately 3.5 ml of oxygen uptake per kilogram body-weight per minute, or 1 kcal per kg body-weight per hour. Thus, as above, a 12 MET activity requires twelve times the metabolic energy expenditure of sitting quietly. By multiplying the body weight in kg by the MET value and the duration of activity one can estimate the energy expenditure that is specific to a person's body weight (one litre of oxygen uptake equals approximately 5 kcal). For example, for a 75 kg person walking 4.7 km/h (appr. 3 METs) for half-an-hour uses 75 x 3 x 0.5 = 112,5 kcal.

CHAPTER 7

A list of MET values for specified activities is published by Ainsworth et al. (1993). However one should be aware of the fact that, for most specified activities other than walking or running, the published MET values are broad estimates representing a whole range of individual intensities. Another problem with the standard MET values is that persons with same body weight may have different energy expenditure during the same activity. Furthermore, external conditions such as wind, surface etc. may affect these values very substantially.

It can be seen that gross inaccuracies of estimate are liable when intensity is given an energy expenditure rating based on generalised calorific equivalents from various sources and total expenditure is then calculated together with the information on frequency and duration.

The most valuable type of information relevant to health considerations is **how strenuously the activity is performed relative to the individual's fitness or capacity**. This will have a bearing on determining which activities are likely to have a beneficial effect on the individual concerned by maintaining or increasing fitness. However, if total energy expenditure is required, albeit as an approximation in population surveys, or by people who are seeking to balance their energy equation to lose body fat or control body weight, then some such means of conversion to kilocalories is the only feasible approach outside the laboratory. Further studies of energy expenditure during activity by normal people are urgently needed.

Other areas of information included in most such questionnaires are
(a) reported medical history
(b) other health related behaviours especially smoking and diet
(c) self appraisal: i.e. perception of relative state of fitness and physical activity
(d) attitude, social influence, self-efficacy-cum-barriers to exercise and exertion
(e) miscellaneous personal details such as socio-economic status, education, position in family

Examples of well-tried questionnaires (but specific to the populations on which they were used) are included in Appendix 4 (Baecke et al. 1982) and 5 (Paffenbarger et al. 1993).

<u>Final Note</u>

While the reliability and precision of the information gained from physical activity questionnaires cannot match that obtained from measurements of physical capacities, the importance of obtaining both cannot be over-emphasised. It is only by having such comprehensive information that associations between lifestyle and health can be examined. Moreover associations which are found in descriptive studies, e.g. a one-off snapshot of the population, can only be analysed for causality in longitudinal studies such as where a cohort approach is used. Monitoring for example of morbidity and mortality, in large population studies, or changes consequent on health interventions, e.g. the effect on a community of exercise promotion, is only possible if the relevant information is obtained in the initial survey.

Assessment of health status

Assessment of health status in conjunction with fitness testing has two main purposes: (1) to ensure the safety of the person being tested and (2) to serve as important supplementary information in exercise guidance based on the fitness assessment.

Similar tests to the Eurofit for Adults battery have already been used quite widely in many countries. When safety aspects have been properly taken into consideration few problems have been encountered. Thus, for safety purposes, all persons who may be subjected to health risks due to the testing should be identified and excluded if the risk is significant. In general all persons in normal health can take the Eurofit tests without risk. However, since many risk factors for disease are widely prevalent in all populations, simple health screening should be part of the testing procedure in order to identify persons at risk. The purpose of such screening is to exclude persons only from those tests that would entail health hazard. Therefore health status may be contraindicative for a certain test or tests but not for all tests. If resources are available, arrangements may sometimes be made for people at risk to perform the tests in the presence of a doctor or nurse.

In exercise counselling the health assessment provides information for safe exercise prescription. Many chronic diseases may limit participation in some types of exercise and

CHAPTER 7

in very strenuous exertion, but many forms of moderate intensity exercise can still be safely practised.

Any severe chronic disease and recent major trauma or surgery may be contraindicative for fitness testing and exercise. Use of medication may introduce limitations or risk to testing and exercising. Acute infection states are temporary contraindications. The health screening is designed to identify the persons at risk and to direct them to proper medical consultation. Pregnancy and recent childbirth, however, being natural healthy states are not in themselves reasons for exclusion from testing or exercise, but will produce results reflecting those conditions.

Since medical policy regulations and practice in connection with sport and physical activity vary greatly between member countries, no strict guidelines for health assessment can be given. Rather, each country should develop its own procedures for this purpose. As an example of such a procedure the Canadian questionnaire (Physical Activity Readiness or PAR-Q) is described below.

The PAR-Q is a self-administered method, which can be used for both screening for testing and for exercise guidance. The original form (Chisholm et al 1975) has been validated by the British Columbia Department of Health (Chisholm et al 1978). It is extensively used in many countries sometimes with minor modifications for both research and exercise promotion purposes. Recently an updated revised version has been introduced (Thomas et al 1992). It comprises seven questions, four additional explanatory notes and the subject's signature, as follows:

PAR-Q questionnaire

1. Has your doctor ever said that you have a heart condition and recommended only medically approved physical activity?

2. Do you have chest pain brought on by physical activity?

3. Have you developed chest pain at rest in the past month?

4. Do you lose consciousness or lose your balance as a result of dizziness?

5. Do you have a bone or joint problem that could be aggravated by the proposed physical activity?

6. Is your doctor currently prescribing medication for your blood pressure or heart condition? (e.g., diuretics or water pills)

7. Are you aware, through your own experience or a doctor's advice, of any other reason against your exercising without medical approval?

Note

1. This questionnaire applies only to those 15 to 69 years of age.

2. If you have temporary illness, such as a fever, or are not feeling well at this time, you may wish to postpone the proposed activity.

3. If you are pregnant, you are advised to discuss the "PAR-X for Pregnancy" form with your physician before exercising.

4. If there are any changes in your status relative to the above questions, please bring this information to the immediate attention of your fitness professional.

I have read, understood and completed this questionnaire.

Signature_____Date_____

Signature of Parent _____or Guardian (for participants under

the age of majority)

Witness_____Date _____

This questionnaire is normally used to exclude all persons having one adverse response. However, the consequence of this in some studies has been to exclude very large percentages of the population being surveyed, these percentages increasing with age. Ideally, the procedure should be used in conjunction with a follow-up examination by a doctor of the implications of the adverse response. In many cases this will result in the person concerned being able to participate, but the correct medical appraisal has then taken place.

References

Ainsworth BE, Haskell WL, Leon AS, Jacobs DR, Montoye HJ, Sallis JF, Paffenbarger RS. 1993. Compendium of physical activities: classification of energy costs of human physical activities. Med Sci Sport Exerc 25(1):71–80.

Baecke SH, Burema O. Frijers JER. 1982. A short questionnaire for the measurement of habitual physical activity in epidemiological studies. Am J Clin Nutr 36:932–942.

Chisholm DM, Collis ML, Kulak LL, Davenport W, Gruber N. 1975. Physical activity readiness. Br Col Med J 17:375–378.

Chisholm DM, Collis ML, Kulak LL, Davenport W, Gruber N, Stewart G. 1978. PAR–Q Validation Report: The evaluation of a self–administered pre–exercise screening questionnaire for adults. Ministry of Health, Vancouver:BC.

Kok GI, Bouter LM. 1990. On the importance of planned health education: prevention of ski–injury as an example. Am J Sports Med 18(6):600–605.

Paffenbarger RS, Blair SN, Lee IM, Hyck RT. 1993. Measurement of physical activity to assess health effects in free–living populations. Med Sci Sports Exerc 25(1):60–71.

Thomas S, Reading J, Shephard RJ. 1992. Revision of the physical activity readiness questionnaire (PAR–Q). Can J Spt Sci 17(4):338–345.

Table 3. Quintile percentage values for maximal aerobic power (mlO_2/kg/min) by age and sex. Swedish population norms[1].

Percentile	Age				
	20-29	30-39	40-49	50-59	60-
Men					
80th	51.6	44.7	39.3	34.8	28.6
60th	45.6	39.4	34.1	31.4	26.4
40th	41.3	34.5	30.9	27.6	23.6
20th	36.2	29.8	27.1	22.5	18.7
Women					
80th	48.2	43.0	38.3	34.0	29.0
60th	43.2	37.9	33.5	29.8	27.2
40th	39.0	34.1	29.5	24.8	23.6
20th	33.6	30.3	25.2	21.8	19.7

[1] Derived from the data of a Swedish national survey. See reference Engström et al. 1993 on p. 84.

TABLES 3-12

Table 4. Quintile percentage values for sit–ups (number of sit–ups) by age and sex. Swedish population norms[1]. (Maximum test result 15 sit–ups.)

Percentile	Age				
	20-29	30-39	40-49	50-59	60-
Men					
80th	15	15	15	15	15
60th	15	15	15	15	15
40th	15	15	15	15	10
20th	15	15	10	8	6
Women					
80th	15	15	15	15	15
60th	15	15	15	13	10
40th	15	15	13	7	6
20th	15	11	6	5	5

[1] Derived from the data of a Swedish national survey. See reference Engström et al. 1993 on p. 84.

Table 5. Quintile percentage values for side-bending (cm) by age and sex. Finnish population norms[1].

Percentile	Age		
	30-39	40-49	50-59
Men			
80th	24.1	23.1	20.6
60th	22.1	21.6	18.7
40th	20.2	19.8	17.1
20th	18.5	15.5	14.7
Women			
80th	23.7	22.5	20.1
60th	21.8	19.9	18.6
40th	21.1	18.6	16.9
20th	17.8	16.1	15.6

[1] Derived from the data of a Finnish study. Urho Kaleva Kekkonen (UKK) Institute for Health Promotion Research & Sports Research Institute of University of Frankfurt (unpublished 1995). FINGER. Finnish-German study on physical activity, fitness and health. Volume 1: Health-related fitness. The assessment methods and descriptive results of common variables in the cross-sectional studies. Tampere: UKK Institute.

TABLES 3-12

Table 6. Quintile percentage values for sit–and–reach (cm) by age and sex. Swedish population norms[1].

Percentile	Age				
	20-29	30-39	40-49	50-59	60-
Men					
80th	40	40	39	35	34
60th	34	34	33	30	29
40th	29	28	27	26	22
20th	20	20	19	18	16
Women					
80th	41	41	39	39	39
60th	36	36	35	34	33
40th	32	31	31	30	29
20th	25	25	25	24	24

[1] Derived from the data of a Swedish national survey. See reference Engström et al. 1993 on p. 84.

Table 7. Quintile percentage values for balance (number of attempts) by age and sex. Swedish population norms[1].

Percentile	Age				
	20-29	30-39	40-49	50-59	60-
Men					
80th	1	1	1	1	2
60th	1	1	2	4	6
40th	1	2	3	4	7
20th	4	6	5	7	11
Women					
80th	1	1	1	2	3
60th	1	1	1	4	6
40th	2	2	3	7	9
20th	4	5	6	10	13

[1] Derived from the data of a Swedish national survey. See reference Engström et al. 1993 on p. 84.

TABLES 3-12

Table 8. Quintile percentage values for vertical jump (cm) by age and sex. Swedish population norms[1].

| Percentile | Age | | | | |
	20-29	30-39	40-49	50-59	60-
Men					
80th	61	55	52	45	39
60th	55	51	47	42	35
40th	52	47	42	37	31
20th	47	42	38	31	24
Women					
80th	43	40	36	30	26
60th	39	35	31	27	23
40th	36	32	28	25	20
20th	31	29	25	21	17

[1] Derived from the data of a Swedish national survey. See reference Engström et al. 1993 on p. 84.

TABLES 3-12

Table 9. Quintile percentage values of shoulder abduction (degrees of rotation) by age and sex. English population norms[1].

| Percentile | Age | | | | |
	20-29	30-39	40-49	50-59	60-65
Men					
80th	164	162	158	152	150
60th	156	154	150	144	140
40th	152	146	144	138	134
20th	144	138	138	130	126
Women					
80th	163	160	156	152	150
60th	156	152	148	144	140
40th	150	146	142	138	132
20th	140	138	134	132	124

Note: It can be seen that up to the age of 65 relatively few individuals will score below the minimal requirement for functional adequacy. However active recreation will often require greater flexibility (see text p. 72).

[1] Derived from the data of an English national survey. See reference The Sports Council and the Health Authority 1992 on p. 35.

TABLES 3-12

Table 10. Quintile percentage values for hand grip strength in relation to body weight (Newtons/kg[1]) by age and sex. English population norms[2].

Percentile	Age				
	20-29	30-39	40-49	50-59	60-65
Men					
80th	8.04	7.91	7.68	7.12	6.66
60th	7.26	7.08	6.71	6.46	6.06
40th	6.60	6.47	6.22	5.89	5.47
20th	5.88	5.55	5.65	5.02	4.97
Women					
80th	5.99	5.84	5.74	5.23	4.73
60th	5.29	5.20	5.09	4.59	4.01
40th	4.83	4.77	4.63	4.02	3.65
20th	4.21	4.04	4.05	3.45	3.15

[1] 1 kg is equivalent to approximately 10 Newtons.
[2] Derived from the data of an English national survey. See reference The Sports Council and the Health Authority 1992 on p. 35.

TABLES 3-12

Table 11. Conversion of the sum of triceps, biceps, subscapula and suprailiac skinfolds to body fatness (body fat as a percentage of weight) (Durnin and Womersley 1974).

Skinfolds (mm)	Males (age in years)				Females (age in years)			
	17–29	30–39	40–49	50+	16–29	30–39	40–49	50+
15	4.8	–	–	–	10.5	–	–	–
20	8.1	12.2	12.2	12.6	14.1	17.0	19.8	21.4
25	10.5	14.2	15.0	15.6	16.8	19.4	22.2	24.0
30	12.9	16.2	17.7	18.6	19.5	21.8	24.5	26.6
35	14.7	17.7	19.6	20.8	21.5	23.7	26.4	28.5
40	16.4	19.2	21.4	22.9	23.4	25.5	28.2	30.3
45	17.7	20.4	23.0	24.7	25.0	26.9	29.6	31.9
50	19.0	21.5	24.6	26.5	26.5	28.2	31.0	33.4
55	20.1	22.5	25.9	27.9	27.8	29.4	32.1	34.6
60	21.2	23.5	27.1	29.2	29.1	30.6	33.2	35.7
65	22.2	24.3	28.2	30.4	30.2	31.6	34.1	36.7
70	23.1	25.1	29.3	31.6	31.2	32.5	35.0	37.7
75	24.0	25.9	30.3	32.7	32.2	33.4	35.9	38.7
80	24.8	26.6	31.2	33.8	33.1	34.3	36.7	39.6
85	25.5	27.2	32.1	34.8	34.0	35.1	37.5	40.4
900	26.2	27.8	33.0	35.8	34.8	35.8	38.3	41.2
95	26.9	28.4	33.7	36.6	35.6	36.5	39.0	41.9
100	27.6	29.0	34.4	37.4	36.4	37.2	39.7	42.6
105	28.2	29.6	35.1	38.2	37.1	37.9	40.4	43.3
110	28.8	30.1	35.8	39.0	37.8	38.6	41.0	43.9
115	29.4	30.6	36.4	39.7	38.4	39.1	41.5	44.5
120	30.0	31.1	37.0	40.4	39.0	39.6	42.0	45.1
125	30.5	31.5	37.6	41.1	39.6	40.1	42.5	45.7
130	31.0	31.9	38.2	41.8	40.2	40.6	43.0	46.2
135	31.5	32.3	38.7	42.4	40.8	41.1	43.5	46.7
140	32.0	32.7	39.2	43.0	41.3	41.6	44.0	47.2
145	32.5	33.1	39.7	43.6	41.8	42.1	44.5	47.7
150	32.9	33.5	40.2	44.1	42.3	42.6	45.0	48.2
155	33.3	33.9	40.7	44.6	42.8	43.1	45.4	48.7
160	33.7	34.3	41.2	45.1	43.3	43.6	45.8	49.2
165	34.1	34.6	41.6	45.6	43.7	44.0	46.2	49.6
170	34.5	34.8	42.0	46.1	44.1	44.4	46.6	50.0
175	34.9	–	–	–	–	44.8	47.0	50.4
180	35.3	–	–	–	–	45.2	47.4	50.8
185	35.6	–	–	–	–	45.6	47.8	51.2
190	35.9	–	–	–	–	45.9	48.2	51.6
195	–	–	–	–	–	46.2	48.5	52.0
200	–	–	–	–	–	46.5	48.8	52.4
205	–	–	–	–	–	–	49.1	52.7
210	–	–	–	–	–	–	49.4	53.0

TABLES 3-12

Table 12. Estimated percent body fat by age for different values of BMI (male). English national survey[1].

Age group	BMI					
	20		25		30	
	Men	Women	Men	Women	Men	Women
16–24	13.0	2.52	20.7	31.2	26.7	36.0
25–34	15.1	25.4	21.3	31.6	26.2	36.5
35–44	18.3	27.9	24.2	33.6	28.9	38.0
45–54	21.2	30.5	27.2	36.1	31.9	40.5
55–64	20.2	32.0	27.5		33.1	41.0

[1] Derived from the data of an English national survey. See reference The Sports Council and the Health Authority 1992 on p. 35.

TABLES 3-12

104

APPENDIX 1

NOTE FROM THE WORKING PARTY

The CDDS Eurofit project started in the late 1970's. It functioned primarily through tri- or biennial Eurofit seminars with frequent informal meetings of a core group of experts. The project first focused on developing a children's fitness test battery. The handbook for the children's Eurofit test battery was first published in 1987 with a subsequent edition in 1993.

On the recommendation of the 6th European research seminar on Eurofit held in Izmair, Turkey, in 1990, CDDS founded a Eurofit coordinating group in 1991 to follow the implementation of the children's Eurofit and to develop a health-related fitness test battery for adults.

Two groups have been responsible for the preparation of the adult Eurofit test battery. The first, the Eurofit Coordinating Group, was established in 1991. The members were:

Hélène Levarlet-Joye	Belgium
Bojidarka Voynska	Bulgaria
Pekka Oja (chairman)	Finland
Eleftherios Tsaruchas	Greece
Aniko Barabás	Hungary
Giuseppe Cilia	Italy
Vida Volbekiene	Lithuania
Willem van Mechelen	The Netherlands
Waldemar Sikorski	Poland
Vadim Balsevich	Russia
Manuel Chamorro	Spain
Juan Antonio Prat	Spain
Björn Ekblom	Sweden
Necatie Akgun	Turkey
Bill Tuxworth	United Kingdom

A working party of the coordinating group, was founded in 1992 to produce the handbook. The members have been Hélène Levarlet-Joye, Pekka Oja (chairman), Aniko Barabás, Willem van Mechelen, Waldemar Sikorski (1992 only), Manuel Chamorro, Björn Ekblom and Bill Tuxworth.

The groups have held the following meetings.

26-27 November 1991, Coordinating Group, Strasbourg

1-2 October 1992, Coordinating Group, Strasbourg

26-27 April 1993, Working Party, Barcelona

20, 23 October 1993, Coordinating Group, Barcelona

21-23 October 1993, 7th Eurofit seminar, Barcelona

16-17 December 1993, Working Party, Amsterdam

27-28 August 1994, Working Party, Budapest

The adult Eurofit handbook has been prepared in the working meetings and through written contributions from the Working Party members. The groundwork was laid in the 1991 and 1992 Coordinating Group's meetings in which presentations on recent or current health-related adult fitness testing were given by the group members.

The aims and objectives of the Eurofit test for adults and the basic structure of the handbook were defined in the 1992 Coordinating Group's meeting. In addition pairs or threesomes of the Working Party members were given writing assignments for the first five chapters. It was foreseen that a provisional handbook could be presented in the 1993 Eurofit seminar.

The structure of the test battery was discussed and tentatively set in the Working Party's meeting in Barcelona in 1993. Additional writing assignments for the last chapter were also given.

The draft version of the handbook was further discussed in the Coordinating Group's meeting in Barcelona and subsequently presented and discussed in the Eurofit seminar. The seminar made several amendments to the handbook and recommended certain changes, which were to be resolved by the Working Party.

At its Amsterdam meeting the Working Party processed the revised version of the provisional handbook. As this meeting was set to be the last for the Working Party, an attempt was made to finalize the draft so that it would be ready for technical editing. This task proved to be impossible due to the fact that the composition of certain tests required further deliberation and a reasonable method for assessing physical activity was not available.

The Working Party has continued its work on the remaining issues during 1994 with the extended support of CDDS. Three members had an informal meeting in connection with an international fitness assessment course in Tampere, Finland, in March. The editors had a working meeting in Tampere August 12-13, 1994. The Working Party met in Budapest August 27-28, 1994 to resolve the remaining substantial issues and to suggest editorial revisions. Handbook-related issues such as the implementation of the test in the member countries, follow-up procedures and possible comparative studies were also discussed and suggestions thereof were made to CDDS. The final meeting of the editorial group was held in Den Burg, Netherlands on November 3-4, 1994. The manuscript was submitted to CDDS in December 1994.

APPENDIX 1

APPENDIX 2

COMMERCIAL EQUIPMENT
FOR FITNESS ASSESSMENT

ANTHROPOMETRIC INSTRUMENTS

Stadiometers (Height)

HOLTAIN Ltd.

Crosswell, Crymmych, Dyfed SA41 3UF, Wales (UK)

Tel. (01239)79656 Fax. (01239)79453

Wall stadiometer (adjustable) (Ref. AW?)

Portable stadiometer (695 - 2078 mm) (Ref. AW 603)

RAVEN EQUIPMENT Ltd.

12 Little Mundells, Welwyn Garden City, Hertfordshire,

AL7 1EW, England. Tel. (01707)320220/Fax (01707)331012

Magnimetre ® wall (0-210 cm) (Ref 503 Scale board/

Ref 504 Detachable measuring arm)

Magnimetre ® freestanding -portable- (0-210 cm) (Ref 503A)

Skinfold calipers

Holtain skinfold caliper (Ref. AW 610) (See address above).

GPM skinfold caliper

Siber Hegner

Pfister Import-Export Inc. 450 Barell Ave., Carltadt; NJ 07072 (USA)

Owl Industries Ltd. 177 Imeda Road, Markham,

Ontario L3R 1A9 (Canada)

Harpenden skinfold caliper

British Indicators Ltd. Quality Houses,

46-56 Dumfries Street, Luton, Beds LU1 5BP (UK)

H.E. Morse Co, 455 Douglas Avenue, Holland MI 49423 (USA)

Harpenden electronic read-out incorporating computer system (HEROICS)

HUMAG Research Group, Department of Human Sciences,

University of Loughborough, Loughborough, Leics. LE11 3TU (UK)

Lafayette skinfold caliper (Ref. LA 01127) (see address below)

Beam scale (weight)

        SECA (Delta model 707 -digital- /model 713 - manual-)

        CMS Weighing Equipment Ltd. 18 Camden High Street, London NW1
OJH, (UK)

        SALTER Weighing Scales. Salter International Measurement Ltd.

        George Street, West Bromwich, Staffs (UK)

        TOLEDO Electronics Scales. Toledo Scale, 431 Ohio Pike,

        Suite 302. Way Cross Office Park, Toledo OH (USA)

FITNESS TESTS

Arm abduction (goniometers)

        LAFAYETTE INSTRUMENT COMPANY

        PO Box 5729. Lafayette, Indiana 47903 USA.

        Tel (317) 423-1505/ Fax. (317) 423-4111

        CAMPDEN INST.

        186 Campden Hill Road, London W8 7TH. UK.

        Tel. 7273437/Fax 2293442.

        MEPSA S.A. Francos Rodriquez 47, 28039 Madrid Spain

        Tel (341)4595289 Fax (341)4595352

Hand Grip

        Hand Dynamometer (model 78010)

        LAFAYETTE INSTRUMENT COMPANY

        (see address above)

Sit-and-reach

        Flexibility tester (Sit and reach box) (Ref. LA 01285)

        LAFAYETTE INSTRUMENT COMPANY

        (see address above)

APPENDIX 2

20-meter shuttle run test

NATIONAL COACHING FOUNDATION

COACHWISE Ltd., 114 Cardigan Road, Headingley, Leeds LS6 3BJ (UK)

Tel. (0532)743889 Fax. (0532)319606

Multistage fitness test (audio casette and booklet) (Ref. AA1)

2 km walking test

Detailed instructions for the organization, conduction and calculations are given in "Guide for the UKK Institute 2-km walking test" (available from: UKK Institute, P.O.Box 30, FIN-33501 Tampere, Finland).

APPENDIX 3

SOUND TRACK CONTENTS FOR THE MULTISTAGE 20 METRE ENDURANCE SHUTTLE RUN WITH STAGES OF 1 MINUTE

A. Location of the test protocol on the tape

'To facilitate location of the various parts of the tape, you hear the countdown: "three, two, one, zero". At zero, set the tape position indicator to "zero". Stand by: "three, two, one, zero"'.

B. Identification of test

'Endurance shuttle test'.

C. Checking tape recorder speed

'Standard calibration period of one minute to check tape recorder speed. Start stopwatch at "go". Stand by. "Three, two, one, go" (set stopwatch in motion)... Stand by for stopping stopwatch: "stop" (stop stopwatch). End of standard calibration period of one minute'.

D. Starting instructions

'The test will start in 30 seconds. Line up at the start. Run for as long as possible, keeping in your lane. Always run in a straight line. If you stop, you stop! - no rests are allowed. When you do stop, note the last number announced for the relevant period - this is your result, so don't forget! The test will start in five seconds' time when the buzzer sounds: 5,4,3,2,1, 'Beep'....beep...beep...
Beginning of stage 1 ...beep...beep...
Stage 2 ... (and so on to stage 21). End of recording'.

NOTE ON THE PROCEDURE FOR RECORDING A SOUND TRACK FOR THE MULTISTAGE 20 METRE SHUTTLE RUN (SEE ALSO TABLE 1).

The use of an electronic recording method is preferable but requires more sophisticated equipment. The manual method is acceptable: even though the chances of error with each sound signal are greater, the margin of error fluctuates and evens out from one signal to the next, the overall effect being practically nil after a two minute period. What matters is systematic error (clock gaining or losing) which should be lower than 1 % (i.e. 0.01 sec).

The information to be recorded will include sections A, B, C, D, from the preceding page, plus the full test protocol outlined at the end of Section D.

Equipment needed:

1. Cassette or reel-to-reel tape recorder (mono or stereo). A 'pause' facility is useful.

2. Microphone.

3. Clock with sweep seconds hand (duration of periods).

4. Manually-operated clock with non-cumulative split timing facility (timing of intervals between sound signals).

or

Electronic clock with adjustable cycles (length of intervals between sound signals.

5. Sound source (electric beeper, whistle, voice). With the electronic method, it must be possible to connect the sound source to the electronic clock. A frequency generator may be used to change the sound frequency from one period to the next.

6. Magnetic tape for a 20 minute recording. 900 foot tape running at 9.5 cm/s (3 3/4 ips) or 45 minutes cassette.

TABLE 1 to Appendix 3. Endurance shuttle run test.

Stage (Minutes)	Speed (km/h)	Split time (Seconds)
1	8,0	9,000
2	8,5	8,000
3	9.0	7,579
4	9.5	7,200
5	10.0	6,858
6	10.5	6,545
7	11.0	6,261
8	11.5	6,000
9	12.0	5,760
10	12.5	5,538
11	13.0	5,333
12	13.5	5,143
13	14.0	4,966
14	14.5	4,800
15	15.0	4,645
16	15.5	4,500
17	16.0	4,364
18	16.5	4,235
19	17.0	4,114
20	17.5	4,000
21	18.0	3,892

TABLE 2 Appendix 3. Shuttle distance adjustment according to cassette player speed. A 60 seconds standard time period is provided. With a stopwatch (accurate to 1/10 sec) check if the duration of the standard time period is actually 60 seconds long. If it is shorter or longer than 60 seconds correct the 20 m running distance using the table.

Standard Time Period (Seconds)	Distance to Run (meters)
55.0	18.333
55.5	18.500
56.0	18.666
56.5	18.833
57.0	19.000
57.5	19.166
58.0	19.333
58.5	19.500
59.0	19.666
59.5	19.833
60.0	20.000
60.5	20.166
61.0	20.333
61.5	20.500
62.0	20.686
62.5	20.833
63.0	21.000
63.5	21.166
64.0	21.333
64.5	21.500
65.0	21.666

CAUTION: With more than a five second error on the standard time period, change the tape player for another one!

APPENDIX 4

Baecke-Questionnaire. codes and method of calculation of index-scores of habitual physical activity.
(For details see reference Baecke et al. 1982 on p. 94)

1) What is your main occupation? (Classified according to occupational physical activity) 1 - 3 - 5
2) At work I sit
   never/seldom/sometimes/often/always 1-2-3-4-5
3) At work I stand
   never/seldom/sometimes/often/always 1-2-3-4-5
4) At work I walk
   never/seldom/sometimes/often/always 1-2-3-4-5
5) At work I lift heavy loads
   never/seldom/sometimes/often/always 1-2-3-4-5
6) After working I am tired
   very often/often/sometimes/seldom/never 5-4-3-2-1
7) At work I sweat
   very often/often/sometimes/seldom/never 5-4-3-2-1
8) In comparison with others of my own age
   I think my work is physically
   much heavier/heavier/as heavy/lighter/much lighter 5-4-3-2-1
9) Do you play sport?
   yes/no

If yes:
- which sport do you play most frequently Intensity 0.76-1.26-1.76 (Mj/h)
- how many hours a week? <1/1-2/2-3/3-4/>4 Time 0.5-1.5-2.5-3.5-4.5
- how many months a year? <1/1-3/4-6/7-9/>9 Proportion 0.04-0.17-0.42-0.67-0.92
If you play a second sport:
- which sport is it? Intensity 0.76-1.26-1.76 (Mj/h)
- how many hours a week? <1/1-2/2-3/3-4/>4 Time 0.5-1.5-2.5-3.5-4.5
- how many months a year? <1/1-3/4-6/7-9/>9 Proportion 0.04-0.17-0.42-0.67-0.92

10) In comparison with others of my own age I think my physical
    activity during leisure time is
    much more/more/the same/less/much less 5-4-3-2-1
11) During leisure time I sweat
    very often/often/sometimes/seldom/never 5-4-3-2-1
12) During leisure time I play sport
    never/seldom/sometimes/often/very often 1-2-3-4-5
13) During leisure time I watch television
    never/seldom/sometimes/often/very often 1-2-3-4-5
14) During leisure time I walk
    never/seldom/sometimes/often/very often 1-2-3-4-5
15) During leisure time I cycle
    never/seldom/sometimes/often/very often 1-2-3-4-5
16) How many minutes do you walk and/or cycle per
    day to and from work, school and shopping?
    <5/5-15/15-30/30-45/>45 1-2-3-4-5

Calculation of the simple sport-score (I_9):
(score of zero is given to people who do not play sport)

$$(I_9): \quad \sum_{i=1}^{2} (\text{Intensity} \times \text{Time} \times \text{Proportion})$$

= 0/0.01-<4/4-<8/8-<12/>12 1-2-3-4-5

Calculation of scores of the indices of physical activity:

WORK INDEX $= \{I_1 + (6-I_2) + I_3 + I_4 + I_5 + I_6 + I_7 + I_8\}/8$

SPORT INDEX $= \{I_9 + I_{10} + I_{11} + I_{12}\}/4$

LEISURE TIME INDEX $= \{(6-I_{13}) + I_{14} + I_{15} + I_{16}\}/4$

Paffenbarger questionnaire

A: Background information

Name _____ Sex _____ Race _____ Date of birth _____ SS#_____
Address _____ Tel. No. _____ 1. Years of school completed _____
2. What is your occupation? _____ 3. If retired, what year? _____
4. Height: _____ feet _____ inches 5. Waist girth: _____ inches 6. Hip girth: _____ inches
7. Weight: _____ pounds 8. What would be a perfect body weight for you? _____ pounds
9. What best represents your outline drawing and weight? (Please record the appropriate drawing number and body weight for each age that applies to you below.)

	No.	Wt.
a. At age 18	____	____
b. At age 25	____	____
c. At age 40	____	____
d. At age 50	____	____
e. At age 60	____	____
f. At age 70	____	____
g. One year ago	____	____
h. Today	____	____

i. Maximum height: _____ feet _____ inches
At age _____
j. Your weight at birth
_____ pounds _____ ounces

10. How many times in your life have you lost the number of pounds shown below?

No. of pounds

No. of times	5	10	20	30	40+
	____	____	____	____	____

B: Past and Present Health Status:

Has a physician ever told you that you have any of the following? (Please check and give year of onset, if applicable.)

	No	Yes	Year of onset		No	Yes	Year of onset
1. Coronary heart disease:				8. Arthritis			
a. Angina pectoris	____	____	____	(Type: _____)	____	____	____
b. Myocardial infarction	____	____	____	9. Osteoporosis	____	____	____
2. Heart arrhytmia	____	____	____	a. Related fractures	____	____	____
3. Stroke	____	____	____	10. Anxiety disorder	____	____	____
4. High blood pressure	____	____	____	11. Depression	____	____	____
5. Diabetes mellitus	____	____	____	12. Cancer	____	____	____
6. Chronic bronchitis	____	____	____	(Site: _____)	____	____	____
7. Chronic back pain	____	____	____	13. Other major diseases	____	____	____
(diagnosis:_____)				(Specify: _____)			

14.
Father's health history
a. Age if alive _____ or b. Age at death _____ c. Cause of death _____

	No	Yes	Age at onset
d. Coronary heart disease	____	____	____
e. Stroke	____	____	____
f. Cancer (Site: _____)	____	____	____

15.
Mother's health history
a. Age if alive _____ or b. Age at death _____ c. Cause of death _____

	No	Yes	Age at onset
d. Coronary heart disease	____	____	____
e. Stroke	____	____	____
f. Cancer (Site: _____)	____	____	____

16.
Women's Reproductive history:

a. Age at menarche _____
b. Oral contraceptive use: ___ No ___ Yes
   Year started_____ Years used _____
c. Postmenopausal hormonens: ___ No ___ Yes
   Year started_____ Years used _____
d. Age at menopause ___
   Natural ___ Artificial___
e. Benign breast disease ___ No ___ Yes

f. Pregnancy

Number	Age	Duration (weeks)	Live-birth	Still-birth	Miscar-riage	Months Infant breastfed
1						
2						
3						
4						

(Pregnancy outcome: Live-birth, Still-birth, Miscarriage)

C: Physical activities :

1. How many city blocks or their equivalent do you regularly walk each day? _____ blocks / day
   (Let 12 blocks = 1 mile.)
2. What is your usual pace of walking? (Please check one.)
   a. ___Casual or strolling (less than 2 mph)   b. ___ Average or normal (2 to 3 mph)
   c. ___ Fairly brisk (3 to 4 mph)   d. ___ Brisk or striding (4 mph or faster)
3. How many flights of stairs do you climb up each day? _____ flights / day (Let 1 flight = 10 steps)
4. List any sports or recreation you have actively participated in during the past year. Please remember seasonal sports or events.

Sport, Recreation, or Other Physical Activity	Number of Times/Year	Average Time/ Episode Hours	Minutes	Years Par-ticipation
a. _____	_____	_____	_____	_____
b. _____	_____	_____	_____	_____
c. _____	_____	_____	_____	_____
d. _____	_____	_____	_____	_____

APPENDIX 5

5. Which of these statements best expresses your wiew? (Please check one)
    a. ___ I take enough exercise to keep healthy. b. ___ I ought to take more exercise. c. ___ Don´t know.
6. At least once a <u>week</u>, do you engage in regular activity akin to brisk walking, jogging, bicycling, swimming, etc.
    long enough to work up a sweat, get your heart thumping, or get out of breath?
    ___ No Why not?_____ ___Yes How many times per week? ___ ___ Activity:_____
7. When you are exercising in your usual fashion, how would you rate your level of exertion (degree of effort)?

0	0,5	1	2	3	4	5	6	7	8	9	10	
Nothing at all	Very very week (just noticeable)	Very weak	Weak	Moderate	Somewhat strong	Strong (heavy)		Very strong			Very very strong (almost maximal)	Maximal

8. On a usual weekday and a weekend day, how much time do you spend on the following activities? Total for each day should add to 24 hours.

	Usual Weekday Hours / Day	Usual Weekend Day Hours / Day
a. Vigorous activity (digging in the garden, strenuous sports, jogging, aerobic dancing, sustained swimming, brisk walking, heavy carpentry, bicycling on hills, etc.)		
b. Moderate activity (housework, light sports, regular walking, golf, yard work, lawn mowing, painting, repairing, light carpentry, ballroom dancing, bicycling on level ground. etc.)		
c. Light activity (office work, driving a car, strolling, personal care, standing with little motion. etc.)		
d. Sitting activity (eating, reading, desk work, watching TV, listening to radio etc.)		
e. Sleeping or reclining		

D. Dietaty and Social Habits
1. How many servings of the following foods do you eat? (Please respond for <u>each</u> food.)

	Almost never	1-3 per month	1-2 per week	3-6 per week	1-2 per day	3-5 per day	6+ per day
			Avarage Use Last Year				
a. Eggs							
b. Whole milk							
c. Low fat milk							
d. Cream							
e. Yogurt							
f. Cheese							
g. Ice cream							
h. Butter							
i. Margarine							
j. Poultry							
k. Fish							
l. Beef, pork, lamb							
m. Vegetables (include potatoes)							
n. Green salads							
o. Breads and cereals							
p. Fruits and fruit juices							
q. Sweet desserts							
r. Candy							
s. Salty snacks							
t. Tea							
u. Coffee							
v. Wine, sherry, port							
w. Beer, ale, stout, etc.							
w. Liquor - whiskey, gin, etc.							

2. How often do you eat in "fast food places" (hamburger, fried chicken, taco, deep-fried food cafes)?
    No. of times per month ___.
3. How often do you eat "TV dinners"? No. of times per month ___.
4. How often are you dieting (eating less than you would like)? (Please check one.)
    a. Never ___. b. Rarely ___. c.Sometimes ___. d. Often ___. e. Always ___.

5. Do you smoke cigarettes now? ___ No ___ Yes How many on an <u>average</u> day? ____ Year started? 19___
6. Did you ever smoke cigarettes? ___ No ___ Yes How many years did you smoke? ____ Year stopped? 19____
7. Do you think a person of your age can do anything to prevent ill health? (Please check one.)
    a. ___ Can definitely do something b. ___ Can perhaps do something c. ___ It is largely a matter of chance.
8. With how many people you have social relationships? (Please insert appropriate numbers.)

Individual	Number	Quality of support					
		None	Weak	Fair	Avarage	Good	Excellent
a. Spouse or family							
b. Friends and fellow workers							
c. Church, club members, etc.							

APPENDIX 5

Coding rules may be obtained by writing to Dr. Paffenbarger.

Sales agents for publications of the Council of Europe
Agents de vente des publications du Conseil de l'Europe

AUSTRALIA/AUSTRALIE
Hunter publications, 58A, Gipps Street
AUS-3066 COLLINGWOOD, Victoria
Fax: (61) 34 19 71 54

AUSTRIA/AUTRICHE
Gerold und Co., Graben 31
A-1011 WIEN 1
Fax: (43) 1512 47 31 29

BELGIUM/BELGIQUE
La Librairie européenne SA
50, avenue A. Jonnart
B-1200 BRUXELLES 20
Fax: (32) 27 35 08 60

Jean de Lannoy
202, avenue du Roi
B-1060 BRUXELLES
Fax: (32) 25 38 08 41

CANADA
Renouf Publishing Company Limited
1294 Algoma Road
CDN-OTTAWA ONT K1B 3W8
Fax: (1) 613 741 54 39

DENMARK/DANEMARK
Munksgaard
PO Box 2148
DK-1016 KØBENHAVN K
Fax: (45) 33 12 93 87

FINLAND/FINLANDE
Akateeminen Kirjakauppa
Keskuskatu 1, PO Box 218
SF-00381 HELSINKI
Fax: (358) 01 21 44 35

GERMANY/ALLEMAGNE
UNO Verlag
Poppelsdorfer Allee 55
D-53115 BONN
Fax: (49) 228 21 74 92

GREECE/GRÈCE
Librairie Kauffmann
Mavrokordatou 9, GR-ATHINAI 106 78
Fax: (30) 13 83 03 20

IRELAND/IRLANDE
Government Stationery Office
4-5 Harcourt Road, IRL-DUBLIN 2
Fax: (353) 14 75 27 60

ISRAEL/ISRAËL
ROY International
PO Box 13056
IL-61130 TEL AVIV
Fax: (972) 349 78 12

ITALY/ITALIE
Libreria Commissionaria Sansoni
Via Duca di Calabria, 1/1
Casella Postale 552, I-50125 FIRENZE
Fax: (39) 55 64 12 57

MALTA/MALTE
L. Sapienza & Sons Ltd
26 Republic Street
PO Box 36
VALLETTA CMR 01
Fax: (356) 246 182

NETHERLANDS/PAYS-BAS
InOr-publikaties, PO Box 202
NL-7480 AE HAAKSBERGEN
Fax: (31) 542 72 92 96

NORWAY/NORVÈGE
Akademika, A/S Universitetsbokhandel
PO Box 84, Blindern
N-0314 OSLO
Fax: (47) 22 85 30 53

PORTUGAL
Livraria Portugal, Rua do Carmo, 70
P-1200 LISBOA
Fax: (351) 13 47 02 64

SPAIN/ESPAGNE
Mundi-Prensa Libros SA
Castelló 37, E-28001 MADRID
Fax: (34) 15 75 39 98

Llibreria de la Generalitat
Rambla dels Estudis, 118
E-08002 BARCELONA
Fax: (34) 34 12 18 54

SWEDEN/SUÈDE
Aktiebolaget CE Fritzes
Regeringsgatan 12, Box 163 56
S-10327 STOCKHOLM
Fax: (46) 821 43 83

SWITZERLAND/SUISSE
Buchhandlung Heinimann & Co.
Kirchgasse 17, CH-8001 ZÜRICH
Fax: (41) 12 51 14 81

BERSY
Route du Manège 60, CP 4040
CH-1950 SION 4
Fax: (41) 27 31 73 32

TURKEY/TURQUIE
Yab-Yay Yayimcilik Sanayi Dagitim Tic Ltd
Barbaros Bulvari 61 Kat 3 Daire 3
Besiktas, TR-ISTANBUL

UNITED KINGDOM/ROYAUME-UNI
HMSO, Agency Section
51 Nine Elms Lane
GB-LONDON SW8 5DR
Fax: (44) 718 73 82 00

**UNITED STATES and CANADA/
ÉTATS-UNIS et CANADA**
Manhattan Publishing Company
468 Albany Post Road
PO Box 850
CROTON-ON-HUDSON, NY 10520, USA
Fax: (1) 914 271 58 56

STRASBOURG
Librairie Kléber
Palais de l'Europe
F-67075 Strasbourg Cedex
Fax: (33) 88 52 91 21

Council of Europe Publishing/Editions du Conseil de l'Europe
Council of Europe/Conseil de l'Europe
F-67075 Strasbourg Cedex
Tel. (33) 88 41 25 81 - Fax (33) 88 41 27 80